"Powerfully and compassionately written, this book re̲ around issues of race, ethnicity, and oppression. Dr. psychology, yoga philosophy, and spiritual activism unity in diversity and of doing the inner work that he̲ .... peppered with captivating stories and opportunities for study through reflection sections, discussion points, and practice. It is a must-read, both for people with privilege and those who experience oppression. It will transform the work of yoga teachers, yoga therapists, psychotherapists, and anyone who wants to be more aware of ethnic and race-based stress and trauma and how to address it."

—*Bo Forbes, PsyD, psychologist, yoga teacher, and author of* Yoga for Emotional Balance

"Dr. Gail Parker has covered the important subject of race-based trauma with sensitivity, scientific precision, and empathy. Yoga is presented with the principles of yoga, detailed practices, convincing case histories, and anecdotes as a way to achieve deep healing. A compelling read for everyone interested in health, healing, and harmony!"

—*Shirley Telles, MBBS, PhD, Director, Patanjali Research Foundation, Haridwar, India*

"Gail Parker has delivered a surprising, thoughtful, rigorous book about how yoga practice can exacerbate racial trauma, especially if it is done without awareness of the unique aspect of race-based stress. Chock full of concise examples and concrete steps, *Restorative Yoga for Ethnic and Race-Based Stress and Trauma* prepares instructors and practitioners alike for the spiritual work of healing racial wounds. This book should be required reading for yoga studio owners, yoga teachers, yoga therapists, and for everyone practicing yoga while black."

—*Desiree Cooper, author, Pulitzer-Prize nominated journalist, and race and gender activist*

"Dr. Parker has gifted the world with this elegant, powerful book of insights, challenges, and hope. She masterfully weaves the worlds of yoga, healing, trauma, and culture in clear, powerful prose. The practices offer you a new understanding of 'yoga'. You aren't addressing the cultural kleshas? Then get the book!"

—*Matthew J. Taylor, PT, PhD, C-IAYT, Director, SmartSafeYoga, past president, IAYT, and international pain and yoga safety expert. www.smartsafeyoga.com*

"We should all be thankful that Gail Parker, wounded by her own experience of racism, stumbled upon a yoga class. Later, as a psychologist, she came to recognize the healing possible in the stillness of Restorative Yoga. This book is Parker's gracious offering, a beautifully written survival guide for those who have experienced ethnic and race-based stress and trauma, but also for those who wound and re-wound others. It demands we be honest and no longer deny or repress our pain or the pain we inflict upon others. It brilliantly shows us that we have the ability to heal and accept with grace the commonness of our humanity."

—*Patrice Gaines, author of* Laughing in the Dark

"A powerful read for people of all races. Dr. Gail Parker insightfully explains the cumulative effects that race based microaggressions and larger traumatic events can have upon the nervous system and state of mind. She weaves together her personal experiences, training as a psychologist, yogic philosophy, and the nurturing practice of restorative yoga to provide a framework for understanding and recovery."

—*Rane Bowen and Jo Stewart, The Flow Artists Podcast*

"A timely, penetrating search for commonality in a racialized world. Dr. Parker expands the construct of trauma as an assault to the fundamental human need to belong and examines the traumatic consequences of social exclusion. Healing requires embracing our inner connectedness and questioning personal and social beliefs that divide us. The book asks more questions than it answers. Let the conversation begin!"

—*Dessa Stone, PhD*

"A transformative book—not just for yoga practitioners. Through yoga philosophy, research, and story Dr. Gail Parker illuminates how we each add to and suffer from racial trauma. The wisdom and practices shared offer the opportunity to heal ourselves and our communities."

—*Helen Avery, yoga teacher and diversity and inclusion journalist*

"Simply put, Dr. Gail Parker's book is an Awakening. Empowering. Inspiring hope. Life-changing!

Dr. Parker offers us a gift of a lifetime! She engages us in a journey into the deep historical underpinnings and progression of racism, and ethnic and race-based trauma, to ground us in an awareness of the enduring visible and invisible 'wounds' to mind, body, emotion, and spirit. She then guides us through, onto a path of HOPE, anchored in the inner work of 'self-study' and the 'healing balm' of Restorative Yoga.

Dr. Parker's in-depth exploration of trauma and its effects…embedded in all our intergenerational lives…made me want to cry. I could identify with the pain, but I was also touched by her care, extraordinary insights, and the wisdom she gives away so generously. Gail Parker speaks from an intuitive and open heart and she will awaken in you a shift of heart and mind that will move you toward the powerful healing potential of a Restorative Yoga practice. Truly life-changing!"

—*Paula Christian Kliger, PhD, psychologist, psychoanalyst,*
organizational consultant, and author of Power Your Heart, You Power
Your Mind: Self-Study then Build a Bridge to Someone *(SEDA Press, 2018)*

"Gail Parker's important work is a welcome portal into a critical conversation in which we are all engaged. Uniquely, this book is also a thoughtful roadmap for furthering that conversation through the healing practices of yoga."

—*Laurie Hyland Robertson, Editor-in-Chief, Yoga Therapy Today*

"Gail Parker has been a trusted colleague for over two decades. I've always admired her ability to keep her finger on the pulse of issues affecting our community. With this book, she combines decades of experience into a guide for yoga teachers and practitioners to transform yoga into an inclusive space for all."

—*Hiram E. Jackson, CEO, Real Times Media*

"Dr. Gail Parker's skills as a psychologist, researcher, yoga educator, and storyteller converge to share multiple ways a comprehensive and practical application of yoga can restore body, mind, and spirit and neutralize the harmful impact of ethnic and race-based stress trauma. She empowers individuals to acknowledge their racial wounding while shining light on the need for deep healing among those who inflict race-based violence. This book is useful for everyone seeking pathways of peace and understanding to heal the human family."

—*Jana Long, Executive Director, Black Yoga Teachers Alliance*

"Dr. Parker has delivered a concise, frank, and yet non-confrontational look into a sensitive subject. She has opened the door for understanding with insightful and gentle provocations that, rather than telling you how to be, encourage beneficial self-reflection and supportive dialogue that can lead to healing. It is not just a book about how the tools of yoga can help heal race-based stress and trauma—it is an invitation to dive into our own psyche and heart, and into the shoes of others—to pierce through the veils of illusion and be able to see clearly. For anyone who has been affected by or contributed to racial prejudices, or perhaps isn't sure, I recommend this book. I also highly recommend this book for any yoga teacher, as it is important to understand where students could be coming from, and how to help support wholeness rather than knowingly or unknowingly contributing to separation and suffering."

—*Serena Jetelina, CYT, Yoga Therapist, and Producer at Yoga International*

"Dr. Gail Parker's *Restorative Yoga for Ethnic and Race-Based Stress and Trauma* is a unique read. Parker writes from the perspective of a woman who grew up during the Jim Crow era—some of America's cruellest, harshest and unjust times.

She is a psychologist. She is a meditation and yoga instructor. All of these experiences create the perfect package to lead this overdue discussion. She is a truth-seeker and wants all of us to find our truth.

This is her gift to us to heal. We all should thank her for guiding us along this path."

—*Regina H. Boone, Photojournalist, Richmond Free Press*

"Our racialized world has wounded not only people of color, but all of us. That is a central message of Gail Parker's book-and why it's such an important one. She invites us to acknowledge our race-based stress and trauma—without shame or blame—then offers compassionate, science-based strategies for healing. It's a needed book in our times."

—*Tamara Jeffries, yoga instructor, Professor of Journalism at Bennett College, former executive editor of Essence magazine*

"This book shook me to my core as I had to not only confront my own trauma as an African-American woman, but the trauma of others. But then it brought me peace (in the form of yoga) as Dr. Gail provided concrete tools for collective healing. If you are committed to any level of social justice, this book is a must read to heal not only yourself but to help heal others."

—*Daheia J. Barr-Anderson, PhD, MSPH, FACSM, 250-hour RYT and conducts research on African-American women*

"Dr. Gail Parker's powerful new book is delivered with love, compassion and liberation. Dr. Parker reminds us, through personal story telling, the wounds and scars caused by racial and ethnic trauma and the need for radical healing. This is the book we have collectively been waiting for. This book is a love offering of straightforward life-changing tools to foster healing in ourselves and transform our communities."

—*Dr. Terry Harris, Co-founder of The Collective STL*

of related interest

The Yoga Teacher Mentor
A Reflective Guide to Holding Spaces, Maintaining
Boundaries, and Creating Inclusive Classes
Jess Glenny
Foreword by Norman Blair
ISBN 978 1 78775 126 2
eISBN 978 1 78775 127 9

Yoga Therapy for Fear
Treating Anxiety, Depression and Rage with the Vagus Nerve and Other Techniques
Beth Spindler
ISBN 978 1 84819 374 1
eISBN 978 0 85701 331 6

Yoga Therapy as a Creative Response to Pain
Matthew J. Taylor
Foreword by John Kepner
ISBN 978 1 84819 356 7
eISBN 978 0 85701 315 6

The Chakras in Grief and Trauma
A Tantric Guide to Energetic Wholeness
Karla Herbert
Illustrated by Rachel Rosenkoetter
ISBN 978 1 84819 365 9
eISBN 978 0 85701 324 8

Trauma-Sensitive Yoga
Dagmar Härle
Foreword by David Emerson
ISBN 978 1 84819 346 8
eISBN 978 0 85701 301 9

RESTORATIVE YOGA FOR ETHNIC AND RACE-BASED STRESS AND TRAUMA

GAIL PARKER, Ph.D.

FOREWORDS BY OCTAVIA F. RAHEEM AND AMY WHEELER, Ph.D.

ILLUSTRATED BY JUSTINE ROSS

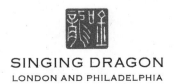

SINGING DRAGON
LONDON AND PHILADELPHIA

First published in Great Britain in 2020 by Singing Dragon,
an imprint of Jessica Kingsley Publishers
An Hachette Company

1

A CIP catalogue record for this title is available from the
British Library and the Library of Congress

ISBN 978 1 78775 185 9
eISBN 978 1 78775 186 6

Printed and bound in the United States

Jessica Kingsley Publishers' policy is to use papers that are natural, renewable and recyclable
products and made from wood grown in sustainable forests. The logging and manufacturing
processes are expected to conform to the environmental regulations of the country of origin.

Jessica Kingsley Publishers
73 Collier Street
London N1 9BE, UK

www.singingdragon.com

This book is for my mother,
Doris Ratliff Parker,
who taught me to always call it as I see it.

CONTENTS

ACKNOWLEDGMENTS

WRITING THIS book has been a labor of love, and birthing it has been hard labor. But, just like birthing a baby, it has been worth it. On top of being hard work, writing a book is all-consuming, with little time for anything else. It has also been a collaborative effort, requiring a team of people, dedicated to supporting, coaching, and advising every step of the way. I could not have done this alone. I want to express my appreciation for and gratitude to my collaborators.

To my husband, Dr. Thomas Walter Johnson, Jr., better known as Tom, Tommy, or T to friends and family. When you retired after a career of dedicated service as a physician, you were so looking forward to spending unlimited amounts of leisure time together, enjoying one another's company, spending time with friends, family, and traveling. As fate would have it, your retirement came just one month before the proposal for this book was accepted, putting a crimp in those plans. So, I start by thanking you first. Throughout this process, you have made tremendous sacrifices by giving me the time alone that was necessary to complete this project. Your unconditional love and support make life so much easier, and make the hard things worth doing. I could not have completed this book without your encouragement, and your unwavering belief in my ability to do it. Thank you for listening to me talk ad infinitum about the book, for leaving me alone to do the writing, for listening to me read to you over and over and over again, and for helping me celebrate victories along the way. You have always shown me what it is to love and be loved. This book is an expression of that. Thank you.

Thank you to my son, Jason Parker Johnson, for making time, in spite of your busy law career, to offer invaluable emotional and I.T. support. You came through with sound advice each and every time I needed an ear to bend and a shoulder to lean on, and with tech support to make this project possible. As much as I needed the I.T. support, your ability to cut to the chase and simplify what I was making unnecessarily complicated streamlined everything. You always calmed my fears when they got in my way. Finally, you have always inspired me to be the best me I can be. ILYMTILY.

To my mother, Doris Ratliff Parker, who wanted to be a professional journalist but, like many women of her generation, was locked out of opportunities to fulfill her potential and who suffered for it. You always claimed that your children were your legacy. I am proud to represent, and I hope I have made you proud. Thank you, Mom.

To my father, Lt. Colonel Frederick Louis Parker, an idealist, who loved to engage in philosophical discussions. I learned so much about life from you, how to dream big and to follow my dreams, and how to make the world a better place. Thank you, Dad.

To my grandmother, Mabel Franklin Ratliff, my mother's mother, the consummate role model of quiet wisdom, strength, courage, and kindness. Your peaceful demeanor was everything, and I thank you for just being you, a role model and a steady non-critical, non-judgmental loving presence in my life. Thank you, Gran.

To my brother, Steven Frederick Parker, your kindness, tenderness, steady support, and humor mean the world to me. You have never let me down and I appreciate you for that. Thank you for always checking in and for always making me laugh, even in times of sorrow; it's a gift and I cherish you for it. Thank you, Steve.

To my friends who held my hand through this process and reassured me that I was on track, or helped me get back on track when I deviated, thank you. Drs. Dessa Stone, Paula Kliger, and Pauline Furman, all of you are great friends, confidants, and amazing psychologists. You gave me advice, sent me research articles, shared stories, and listened as I sorted out my own thoughts during the writing process. To keep me from going off the deep end, you offered some great psychological counseling when I needed it. Writing a book can take you to the edge sometimes. Thank you for being there.

To my yoga family, where do I begin? Thank you to Oliver Black, Yogacharya, my first ever yoga teacher who introduced me to the practice in a way that made me fall in love with it forever.

Thank you to Veronica Zador. You introduced me to Restorative Yoga, taught me how to teach it, and brought me on board as faculty to teach in the Beaumont School of Yoga Therapy. I am forever grateful. I love you as a teacher, a colleague, and a friend.

Thank you, Octavia F. Raheem, Co-Owner of Sacred Chill {West} in Atlanta, for your friendship, for your support of my work from the very beginning, and for sharing your wisdom by writing a beautiful, heartfelt foreword. The creation and use of the illustrations in this book are the result of a seed you planted years ago, requesting a book with images in it that look like us. Your generosity of spirit and unwavering support are priceless.

Thank you, Dr. Amy Wheeler, President of the International Association of Yoga Therapists, and founder of The Optimal State Certified Yoga Therapist Training, for sharing your experience of this work by writing a foreword from a deeply personal perspective. I admire your willingness to speak from a place of such vulnerability. Thank you for your openness, warmth, and friendship. Finally, thank you for being steadfast in your support of this work by faithfully doing your own inner work, attending workshops, participating in webinars, and for introducing this work in your yoga therapy training.

Thank you, Jana Long, Executive Director of the Black Yoga Teachers Alliance (BYTA), and Maya Breuer, Vice President of Cross-Cultural Advancement at Yoga Alliance, two visionaries, for inviting me to present this work at both the inaugural and the second Black Yoga Teachers Alliance Conference at the Kripalu Center for Health. Thank you both for founding BYTA, an alliance that supports the educational and professional development of Black yoga teachers, and offers a platform for those who teach and practice, especially in communities that have traditionally had limited or no access to the practice.

Thank you to Tamara Jeffries, an Advisory Board member of BYTA, and professor of journalism at Bennett College, for your editorial expertise, starting with reading and then offering feedback on the book proposal. I know it was accepted because of your input.

Thank you to Pamela Stokes Eggleston and Amina Naru, Co-Executive Directors of the Yoga Service Council, for championing this work and for promoting it through the webinar series, *Yoga from the Inside Out: Shining a Light on Racial Wounding*. Our monthly consults regarding that project blossomed into friendship and helped me clarify my ideas about how this information should be presented in book form, plus talking to you every month in the process of creating the webinar series was lots of fun.

Todd Tesen is the friend and yoga teacher I mention in the book who helped me heal my back through Restorative Yoga when I fell. Thank you, Todd, for your friendship, for your masterful teaching, for creating welcoming and safe holding environments, and for making the study and practice of yoga such a delight.

Thank you to Jaye Sanders, a faithful student of yoga, for consistently but gently urging me to write, and for generously offering and sharing your encouragement. Thank you for asking Justine Ross to create the beautiful illustrations in this book, and thank you, Justine, for your beautiful artwork.

Thank you to Danielle Graham, my trusted and invaluable assistant, who appeared like a gift from heaven at just the right time to help format and take the fear out of the technical aspects of putting the manuscript together and preparing to send it to the publisher. When you told me not to worry about any of that, and to just concentrate on writing, my life changed for the better.

Thank you, Eddie Stern, for your interest in this work, for your friendship, for your support before, during, and after the writing process, and for gazing over my shoulder with non-critical, loving eyes as I wrote.

Thank you to author Patrice Gaines for your wisdom, humor, and great advice about how to approach writer's block through meditation. It works!

Thank you, of course, to everyone who contributed a part of your story, bringing to life the power of these practices to repair, restore, and recover from deep emotional wounds, and for your courageous efforts to shine a light on the need for this work. Thank you to those who recognize the devastating impact of ethnic and race-based stress and trauma on all of us, in particular to Terry and Ericka Harris and The Collective, and Laura Humpf, who understand and utilize yoga as a strategy for healing the wounds of ethnic and racial distress.

Thank you to Michelle Saahene and Melissa DePino, founders of From Privilege to Progress, for actively engaging in doing work to change hearts and minds by reminding us that it is our shared humanity that counts the most.

Thank you to John Kepner for inviting me to submit a proposal to present at the Symposium of Yoga Therapy and Research (SYTAR) in

2017, and to the Board of the International Association of Yoga Therapists (IAYT) for welcoming me back the following year to be a plenary speaker and workshop presenter. Without knowing that it would, your invitations got the ball rolling on this writing project. Thank you to Matt Taylor, past president of IAYT, for taking time to answer my questions and offer advice about the publishing process.

Thank you to Claire Wilson, Senior Commissioning Editor at Singing Dragon, for inviting me to write this book; to Singing Dragon for accepting the book proposal and for publishing the book; and to Sarah Hamlin, Commissioning Editor at Singing Dragon, for always answering my questions immediately, for your belief in the importance of this work, and for your patience and encouragement throughout this process.

NOTE

The anecdotes, case studies, and interviews included in this book are from my own experience, from the experience of students, clients, colleagues, friends, family, and those actively involved in social justice. Some have given permission to use their names; others have asked that their names be changed. Some of the stories have been combined with others to protect identities. Each story has been thoughtfully selected as representative of experiences that illustrate some of the pain and suffering people have endured as a result of ethnic and race-based stress and trauma, and of Restorative Yoga's potential to alleviate some of the distress.

FOREWORD

OCTAVIA F. RAHEEM

I WILL never forget when I first met Dr. Gail Parker. I noticed something. Her shoulders were relaxed and down. Wholeness, a kind of ease, even grace radiated from the center of her chest. I was struck by the lift in her heart. I was a yoga teacher and in my early 30s, yet I had rarely encountered a woman who moved with such lightness emanating from her heart.

Earlier that same year my mother had survived a type of heart attack that her surgeon said many people do not. Of course, there are many factors, some would call them "lifestyle," yet who can tally the impact of decades of race-based stress and trauma on my mother's heart? How long had she been under pressure? Did it start the day she was born, or in her mother's womb? What really attacked her heart? Who's counting the additional weight of each negative race-based experience? Could the sum of it lead to a broken heart that fights against itself?

I met Dr. Parker at the Yoga Retreat for Women of Color™ led by Maya Breuer in 2012. We "randomly" partnered for an exercise that required us to sit face to face, knee to knee, heart to heart, and speak our truth. From the moment I sat in front of Gail, I felt seen. Even before I opened my mouth, I knew she heard more than I could ever say. I learned later that she was a psychotherapist, meditation and Restorative Yoga teacher, and mother. I am sure the knowledge, skill, and wisdom she's earned in those roles greatly contribute to her capacity to be so present. I also believe there is something else, a subtler quality and energy that I experienced in that moment: The compassion and permission that are wordlessly granted when we are in the presence of someone whose heart has been broken by the world, yet they've been able to recover their wholeness.

I once read that when Dr. King was examined post death, he was found to have the heart of a 65-year-old. He was only 39. To say his heart was heavy and weary is an understatement. To say it was weighted is to misstate the magnitude of the load. It doesn't diminish his legacy or his battle for human and civil rights for all, if we, for this singular moment, ponder the impact only race had on the sustained wear and tear within his heart. Who can calculate the ways that the stress and trauma of racism clog one's arteries, creating blockages and inhibiting access to deeper inner movement?

In 2016 I had the opportunity to formally study Restorative Yoga in a teacher training format led by Dr. Parker. Having studied Restorative Yoga in many different capacities, I was delighted to continue my learning with Gail. The first night of training we discussed stress responses. Previous restorative trainings I had attended only examined the fight-or-flight response. Gail included another response, tend and befriend, a uniquely feminine response to stress first proposed by Shelley E. Taylor. That inclusion of what is often left out of Restorative Yoga training's initial overview of the stress response was a prelude to the way Dr. Parker taught Restorative Yoga and trained teachers: As only a woman with 50+ years of experience as a psychologist, researcher, community leader, *in addition* to yoga educator/therapist could.

Over the course of that first Restorative Yoga teacher training with Gail she addressed something else I'd never heard acknowledged in all of my years of being a student and teacher of yoga—*race-based trauma and stress*. Within her naming of this, I found affirmation of so much of my experience as an African American woman in the world. She offered the perspective that teachers of yoga need to first be aware of this stress and impact within self in order to be more aware of it within our students. That training was the first time I realized that I could more deliberately use Restorative Yoga as a tool to support me in some of my biggest areas of challenge and ongoing stress—those due to race. I knew that this work and the lens through which Dr. Parker offered it could radically change an individual's relationship to self. The trajectory of my work as a yoga teacher shifted. Later that year I opened a yoga studio, Sacred Chill {West}, and decided to focus on Restorative Yoga and yoga styles that are more easeful in nature—meditation and Yoga Nidra.

Sometimes I lay my head against my husband's chest and listen to the life story it taps out. Sometimes it drums rapidly and full of strained whispers, running, running, running. I wonder what memory, experience, or recent encounter in his skin is calling out through his elevated pulse when I hear that frantic banging from the door of his heart?

In 2017, I had the opportunity to be a yoga student in Dr. Parker's immersion—Restorative Yoga for Resilience: Bouncing Back from Race-Based Trauma and Stress for People of Color, in Atlanta, Georgia. Individuals traveled from as far as Boston and the Bahamas to attend. The room was full of yoga teachers, maternal and mental health specialists, professors, public and private educators, corporate executives—a wide range of individuals who'd heard about Gail's work and needed to experience it for themselves. The immersion wasn't about learning how to teach Restorative Yoga; it was about using it to intentionally cultivate a tool for self-care and to manage the stress and trauma that arise from the daily lived experiences as a person of color.

In that immersion I finally had the space and courage to fully recall sitting in my 9th-grade class in front of a young White man who thought it was funny to tap me on the head and call me the "n" word whenever the teacher wasn't looking. I remembered how I chose silence and not speaking up for myself (for weeks) because I feared no one would believe me if I told them what was happening. I remembered deciding I'd had enough and leaving the class with no explanation. I went straight to my counselor and told her what was happening and how it made me feel unsafe and distracted me from learning. My counselor asked me if I was sure that what he was saying was the "n" word… *I did say it was a whisper, didn't I?* I remembered how nothing happened to the young man. Despite the sinking feeling that I felt in that classroom and school from that point forward, I went through the rest of that school year convincing myself I didn't hear what I heard or feel what I felt. That I must have made it all up.

In her immersion, Gail asked me where I felt that experience in my body when I shared the story. My chest tightened. My breath became shallow. I felt exactly the place in my heart that had been broken from that 9th-grade encounter. In that immersion we didn't only tell our stories without the threat of penalty or recourse, which in and of itself was sacred elixir; we applied the balm of Restorative Yoga. We were held in supported postures. We were invited to rest and feel. Rest and release. Rest and allow. Rest and know that we didn't cause the wound, yet it exists. By the end of that immersive experience and being held in such deep truth, community, and compassion, that place of separation and pain in my heart was indeed the place that "light" had entered. I left knowing a way to be more whole.

I recently asked my three-year-old son where his heart was and he touched my chest and said, "In there," and then he touched his own chest, and said, "Here too, Mama." He smiled.

I wonder if he meant his heart feels all of the living, age, time, and experiences of mine?

If his heart is already stronger than other little boys' because of it.

I thought of Gail's heart and the radiance coming from within it.

I thought of my mother's heart.

I thought of Dr. King's old heart in that young body.

I thought of my husband's heart.

I thought of our individual and collective hearts and all of the ways we've been broken.

Through tears I still smiled.

Through Dr. Gail Parker's work and this book, I know a way to restore a sense of wholeness within my heart and myself. I have that wholeness to offer my son and our beloved world.

Octavia F. Raheem
Co-Owner, Sacred Chill {West}
Atlanta, Georgia
October 2019

FOREWORD

AMY WHEELER, PH.D.

GAIL PARKER has opened my eyes and my heart to the issue of race-based traumatic stress and how yoga can help each one of us to heal from the inside out.

My first personal experience with Gail was at a workshop at the Symposium of Yoga Therapy and Research (SYTAR) in 2018. I saw that I was assigned to introduce Gail Parker and that she had chosen to talk about the topic of race-based stress and trauma. My heart skipped a beat. This talk was something very new and exciting, and had never been done before at a SYTAR conference.

Gail gave a short introduction to start the workshop, and then we broke into partners to have a discussion. We were asked to share with our partner about the first time each of us remembered having an awareness of our own race, the race of another person, and the experience, perception, and feelings that came up for us during these early exposures. Some of these early experiences had caused deep emotional imprints in our hearts. I bonded with my new Indian friend during the workshop experience, and we are still in touch today! In those precious moments I felt that I had gained a very small glimpse into the heart of another. I could see the pain inside of my new friend, and was able to imagine how it felt to be judged partially or solely because of one's skin color. During this workshop, I was also able to examine my own feelings and reactions to race and racism, and I began to notice what was churning inside of me during and after the conversation. I realized that people who have direct experiences of negative race-related events need opportunities to recover from the ongoing stress and traumas they experience over a lifetime.

I came away realizing how important it is for yoga teachers and yoga therapists to understand the impact of race-based stress and trauma as they work with students and clients.

Fast forward and I was teaching at my own yoga therapy school. I was feeling confident that it was time for our yoga therapists in training to learn about race-based stress and trauma, its impact on people, and how yoga therapy might be a method to help clients find wholeness again. I felt I had done the research, talked to experts in the field of race relations, and I had learned from Gail in her online course *Yoga from the Inside Out: Shining a Light on Racial Wounding*. I was the daughter of civil rights activists, and felt I was made for this moment in time. I thought to myself, "Be gentle with yourself and others, role-model the ability to give empathy as needed, pause and listen with openness and receptivity...you got this!"

Simply put, I underestimated the task at hand. It is not as easy as Gail makes it look.

I did not understand the gravity of what I was about to take on and how many people in the room had deep trauma around race and racism. I quickly found out that it doesn't matter what color your skin is, or what race or ethnicity one is. We have all been affected. It does not matter if you are the receiver of injustice, the perpetrator of injustice, or just a clueless person who is not keeping up with the social issues of the 21st century. I think that we as individuals, and as a society, have deep wounding around these issues, both consciously and unconsciously.

During that yoga therapy training, our community had experienced several days of group trust, compassion, and kindness. But suddenly our emotionally safe classroom turned into a large emotion-filled brushfire, and tears were shed all around. In the end, we stopped the discussion because it was too painful for all involved. And that was the end of my first attempt to help our group understand one another's feelings, reactions, and nervous system arousal around the issues of race, racism, trauma, and stress. But it will not be my last attempt. I feel that we are all responsible to continue to learn and stretch our edges around this topic.

I am committed to working with Gail to spread her message. Gail's message is one of hope, and faith and courage. She teaches us that each one of us has the ability to go inward and study ourselves, to notice our reactions, our emotions, our thoughts, and our words. We can begin to understand how our own nervous system uniquely functions in times of stress, especially when approaching topics of race and racism. Gail suggests that the pathway forward is by using the tools of Restorative Yoga, self-reflection, and sharing our stories with each other from a place of self-reflective awareness. The work is an inside job for each person. The inner softening will occur over a period of time, with large amounts of commitment, patience, and self-compassion.

I believe that yoga therapy has tremendous potential to help alleviate the pain and suffering of race-based stress and trauma. Even though ethnic and racial injuries have not been studied often or well in the scientific literature, I believe that the field of yoga therapy is uniquely positioned to take the lead in making a significant contribution to studying and delivering specific yoga and meditation practices, within a racially and culturally informed context, that can aid in recovery from race-based stress and trauma. But therapists must first be educated about the unique nature of race-based traumatic stress, the context in which it occurs, and the therapeutic interventions that are appropriate. They must also learn to deal with their own issues around race and ethnicity in order to be effective working with clients.

I hope that you will join Gail by reading and contemplating this significant offering to this world. Get ready to experience the revolution of your own heart. Like me, you may have thought that you were already well on the path of gaining more wisdom in this area. I guarantee this book will make you take a second look at your own mind and heart, your relationship to the people you love and your community. I challenge you to allow the suffering around race and racism to wash over you and through you, so that each of us can make progress towards healing the trauma we are all holding together.

Amy Wheeler, Ph.D.
President, IAYT
October 2019

PREFACE

UNTIL NOW, ethnic and race-based traumatic stress has been a neglected area of inquiry in most trauma-informed therapeutic modalities, including trauma-informed yoga. Yet many of us working in the field of stress reduction and trauma recovery, and those of us living the reality, recognize it as a real and unique source of emotional injury. As a psychologist, a major concern of mine is that ignoring ethnic and race-based stress and trauma as realities can, and I suspect does, run the risk of re-traumatizing people and interferes with the ability to derive maximum benefit from therapeutic intervention and yoga practices in general.

My original intention was to limit sharing my interest in Restorative Yoga as a self-care strategy for race-based stress and trauma with yoga teachers, practitioners, and therapists who have been directly impacted by racial stress and trauma, those who need these practices the most. In all honesty I did not think it would be a topic of interest to anyone else. But as word of my work spread, I began to receive invitations to offer presentations, webinars, and workshops to yoga students, teachers and therapists, medical professionals, and behavioral health professionals, regardless of race and ethnicity, who are interested in learning more.

In 2017 John Kepner, the Executive Director of the International Association of Yoga Therapists (IAYT), invited me to submit a proposal to share my work at the organization's yearly Symposium of Yoga Therapy and Research (SYTAR) conference. The proposal was accepted and the presentation I offered was so well received that I was invited back the following year as a plenary speaker and workshop presenter. Immediately following the 2018 SYTAR conference, Claire Wilson, Senior Commissioning Editor at Singing Dragon, who was in attendance, asked if I would be interested in writing a book on the topic. I said yes, submitted a proposal that was accepted, and this is how *Restorative Yoga for Ethnic and Race-Based Stress and Trauma* was conceived. At the same conference I was approached by Pamela Stokes Eggleston and Amina Naru, Co-Executive Directors of the Yoga Service Council, who asked me to create and facilitate a six-module webinar on the topic of Restorative Yoga for racial stress and trauma. In 2019, *Yoga from the Inside Out: Healing the Wounds of Racial Distress* was born. That same year I was invited to speak on the topic at the 2019 Yoga and Science Conference, held at New York University, hosted by Eddie Stern and Marshall Hagins. I shared the program with Drs. Deepak Chopra, Stephen Porges, Shirley Telles, Sat Bir Khalsa, and other pre-eminent researchers in the field.

I was hesitant at first to step outside my comfort zone and share my thoughts, insights, and understanding with racially mixed groups of people, because of the complexity associated with engaging in this emotionally charged topic cross-racially. But with the support and encouragement of my husband and son, friends, and colleagues of all races and ethnicities, plus my own determination not to let my fears and vulnerabilities stop me, I found the courage to address the issue with any and all who have an interest in learning about the potential for Restorative Yoga, taught within a culturally and racially informed context, to contribute to the alleviation of the pain and suffering of ethnic and race-based stress and trauma.

In addition to the workshops and presentations I offer, I am a faculty member in the Beaumont School of Yoga Therapy, the only hospital-based school of yoga therapy in the United States. I teach yoga teachers who aspire to be yoga therapists how to utilize yoga as a therapeutic strategy to relieve stress and recover from trauma, and to support emotional balance and psychological well-being. Part of my teaching has always focused on the importance of the therapeutic relationship as the container for transformational change in patients.

Following a lecture I gave regarding race-based stress and trauma to aspiring yoga therapists, a student wrote in her evaluation of the class: "I feel most people, not ethnic or of color, do not understand the racial stress talk. They get uncomfortable; an exercise might better help give an idea as to what it feels like to be discriminated against." What stood out most for me was the assertion that "most people, not ethnic or of color" do not understand what it feels like to be discriminated against. The student's feedback reminded me that racial wounding hides in the shadows, and unless and until we shine a light on it, first within ourselves, there is no possibility of lasting change and there is a real possibility of re-wounding and re-traumatizing that can and does occur. This book is an invitation to shine that light first and foremost on ourselves. This is yoga from the inside out.

INTRODUCTION

RACE MATTERS

It is my observation that in a racialized world, each of us has emotional wounds based on events of ethnic and race-based stress and trauma that are unacknowledged and therefore unhealed. Even though visible and invisible effects of ethnic and racial stress and trauma abound, many of us remain unaware of its effects because it is so common. The challenge of doing the hard work of healing the ancient pain of racial wounding is long overdue. It is time for each one of us to take an honest look at the wounding we have endured, and the wounding we have inflicted on others, whether intentional or not. We hurt others as a result of ignorance and of our own inner strife and pain. Now is a time for us to turn within and for healing our own pain as if our very lives depended on it because they do. I believe Restorative Yoga is a tool that can help us do that.

It is time for truth and reconciliation. We don't need to wait for a commission to be formed, or for systems and other individuals to change in order to do this work. This is an inside job. The work I'm talking about is personal. We can begin the process ourselves. In order to effect social change, we have to approach the task of educating ourselves and of healing our internal wounds with courage, dedication, and devotion. But the work we have to do goes beyond policy changes, diversity and inclusion initiatives, and laws. The work we have to do requires shifts in consciousness and it starts with individual personal transformation. No law or policy can make that happen. It is time to shine a light on our own ethnic and racial wounds and to begin the process of healing ourselves. This new revolution is going to be internalized, not broadcast or televised. Now is a time for a change of heart, change that occurs from the inside out.

Restorative Yoga for Ethnic and Race-Based Stress and Trauma is unique because it invites people of all races, ethnicities, cultures, and nationalities to examine how living in a racialized world affects each of us: from the stress and trauma of the daily lived experiences of racial wounding that people endure, to 'White fragility'—"a state in which even a minimum amount of racial stress becomes intolerable, triggering a range of defensive reactions" (DiAngelo 2011, p.57). This book is intended to be a guide for all who are ready to do the work.

Racialized attitudes and adherence to racial stereotypes within the yoga community of practitioners, teachers, and therapists have the potential to negatively impact the quality of the experience of the students taking classes and the patients involved in yoga therapy. When yoga teachers, educators, and therapists lack critical awareness of race and racism, and have not adequately dealt with their own racial hang-ups, which I regard as a symptom of unhealed racial wounds, and when they are uncomfortable and unprepared to deal with issues of race as they come up, they become part of the problem. Yoga teaches us to learn through experiential rather than through theoretical or empirical evidence. This, as far as I am concerned, makes the yoga community an ideal container for constructive conversations about race and ethnicity because talking about race and ethnicity is about telling your story and validating your own lived experience.

We are all affected by race and ethnicity, and it begins in childhood. A look at the seminal work of American psychologists Mamie and Kenneth Clark and educator Jane Elliott points out what living in a racialized culture feels and looks like, and what impact it has on children regardless of race and ethnicity.

In the 1940s the Clarks conducted research to determine how racial segregation affected African American children's attitudes about themselves in particular and about race in general. In an experiment, African American elementary school children were asked to choose between playing with a white-skinned or a brown-skinned doll, to identify which doll they thought was good or bad, and which doll they thought looked most like them. Most of the children preferred the white-toned doll and associated it with being good and associated the brown-toned doll with being bad. Some of the children would cry and run out of the room when asked to identify which doll looked most like them. The results showed how color barriers harmed African American children and helped push the United States Supreme Court to outlaw segregated schools (Blakemore 2018).

The Clarks' experiment was replicated and then reported in 2010, by University of Chicago professor and child psychologist Margaret Beale Spencer, only this time both Black and White children were included. The children were given two sets of cards each, with images of people or animal characters ranging in skin colors from dark to light. Phase one of the study found that the children in each group selected the white images as preferable 70 to 80 percent of the time, reflecting strong bias toward the white images and negative beliefs around the dark images, but the White children showed a significantly stronger bias toward the white images than the Black children. The second phase of the study showed that the preferences of the children to see white as good and black as bad could be modified when they were rewarded for choosing the dark-skinned images over the light-skinned images, demonstrating that their preferences were learned, and under the right conditions could be unlearned (UChicago Magazine 2010).

In 1968, the day after Martin Luther King Jr. was assassinated, Jane Elliott conducted an experiment with her third-grade class to give them the experience of what it is like to be discriminated against. Because they all shared similar skin color, she chose eye color as the thing that set them apart from each other. One day the brown-eyed children were considered superior and the next day the blue-eyed children were considered superior. A documentary film called *The Eye of the Storm* (Elliott 2017[1970]) shows the lesson in discrimination she taught her students. It shows the effects of discrimination on the children, how it transformed them and how they reacted. When they were in the superior group, the children became aggressive, hostile, and dismissive toward those in the inferior group. When they were in the inferior group, the children became sad, confused, and withdrawn, and by the end of the day looked defeated.

All of the children understood that non-White people were treated as if they were inferior to White people. What they did not know was how it felt to regard oneself as being superior and how it felt to be treated as if they were inferior. During that experiment they learned. In a follow-up documentary called *A Class Divided* (Peters 1985), the third-grade students returned as adults to see the first video and to discuss how they had been impacted by the original experiment. They all said it was life-changing.

Each of us has our own unique response to the stress and trauma of ethnic and racial insensitivity, discrimination, injustice, hostility, and violence. Each of us has our own unique way of recovering. Rather than remaining on the surface of ethnic and racial wounding and treating the symptoms of race-based stress and trauma by trying to ignore it, cover it up, fix it, or fight it, what if, instead, we began to contemplate our own experiences of ethnicity and race, including how we have been hurt and how we have been hurtful, and then shared our stories with each other? Addressing our own experiences of racial wounding, including the inability to empathize with or talk non-defensively about race, is key to understanding our responses to race and ethnicity, and can unlock the secrets to healing the wounds of race-based stress and trauma.

You cannot be effective with others unless you have explored your own inner dynamics regarding race and ethnicity. This inner exploration is ongoing and not something you do once and for all. As long as we live in a racialized world, you will need to revisit this exploration time and time again. This book is an invitation to go deeper into this exploration than you may have ever gone before. It is intended to be as much about self-study and self-care as it is about working with others to alleviate the wounds of racial distress.

An important step in easing the suffering associated with ethnic and race-based stress and trauma requires a willingness to share our stories with each other. I will begin with my own. Beginning here is not intended to ignore or exclude the history or ethnic and racial context of others; rather, it is to encourage readers to consider how your own racial, ethnic, and cultural context and your place in history influence your experiences and perceptions of race and ethnicity, stress and trauma. Context matters. Because of my personal context, most of the examples I use and references I make throughout the book are based on my experiences as an African American; however, the examples I cite and the reactions to events of ethnic and racial discrimination and harassment can be applied universally.

MY STORY

Middle school seems to be a time when children separate out socially along racial lines. This was certainly true in my case. I knew about racial prejudice because my parents had taught me about it, but my firsthand experience of it came in sixth grade. We were given an assignment to trace our cultural lineage, show it geographically on a map, and then to report about it in class. I remember being really excited and proud to share what I had learned from my parents and grandparents, especially about my African heritage. When I read my report to the class, they burst out laughing when I mentioned Africa, and began to imitate monkey faces, gestures, and sounds. I remember feeling flushed with embarrassment.

My next memory of other people's reactions to race came later that same year. Our teacher was committed to teaching us social skills, including good manners, ballroom dancing, and dating protocols. Remember, this was a long time ago. Each boy in the class was expected to ask a girl in the class to accompany him to a pre-arranged, chaperoned school dance. When I was asked to go to the dance, I was excited in only the way a pre-pubescent eleven-year-old girl can be. On the evening of the dance, the boy who asked me, and his father, showed up at my house at the appointed time. He gave me a wrist corsage, as our teacher had instructed. Needless to say, I felt very grown up. After our parents introduced themselves to each other, the boy, his father, and I got in the car and off to the dance we went. The rest of the evening was a blur, but I remember having a good time. We won the ballroom dance contest and we each got a little trophy. I was really proud to show it to my parents when I got home.

The day after the dance, I arrived at school and took my seat as usual. I didn't know exactly what it was, but something felt different as soon as I sat down. It wasn't until recess that I realized no one was looking at me, talking to me, or playing with me, and when I approached, they would turn their backs or run away, including my best friend since second grade. Overnight, I had become an outcast. To this day, I am at a loss for words to describe how that felt. Some pain can only be experienced, not explained. Being ostracized continued for the rest of the school year.

At the time we were a military family living on a military base. Even though the Armed Forces were no longer segregated, racism was still a part of military culture, and segregation was still the law in the state where we lived. Interracial dating was not accepted, and interracial marriage was still prohibited by law in the United States. This was during a time of upheaval in America's history when desegregation forces were threatening the status quo of White racial superiority. Images on nightly television news reports, showing the fear and hatred in the faces of those opposed to desegregation, were constant. Given the times, it is likely that someone said something after the school dance that resulted in my classmates treating me the way they did for the remainder of the school year.

For some reason, I never told my parents what happened that day. Eventually, though, my mother could tell that something was terribly wrong. I had become quiet and withdrawn and kept to myself after school. When she asked me why I wasn't playing with my friends, I just shrugged my shoulders and said I didn't want to. But she intuitively connected the dots and realized what was happening. Out of a need to protect my brother and me from the cruelty they knew we were facing, my parents decided that my mother would no longer travel with my father and would instead return with us to her hometown and raise us there. Without much warning or explanation, at the beginning of my seventh-grade year, we left the place we had lived for five years, a long time for a military family, and we were plopped down into a large metropolitan area. My father did not live with us for another two years. He went to Vietnam.

Without any explanation, without anyone to talk to about my feelings of being uprooted from a place I loved and called home, missing my father, missing my friends, still stinging from the pain of rejection, all I could feel was sad and lost. I couldn't talk to my mother because she was too worried about my father, so I kept everything inside and adjusted to my new reality. The elephant in the room, the thing that was never discussed, was the impact of the social exclusion I had experienced. With no adult input to support a more informed perspective, I concluded, as many children might, that there was something wrong with me. My understanding that it was not me came much later. I have often wondered what the impact of shunning me had on my classmates. Did they know how hurtful their behavior was? Did they know why they were doing it? Do they even remember it?

I came of age during the Civil Rights, Black Power, and Black is Beautiful cultural movements in the 1960s and 1970s. The goals of these movements included ending racial discrimination and segregation, promoting self-advocacy, and undoing the cruel legacy of enslavement that erased African culture and that regarded African bodies as unattractive and only suitable for slave labor. We were Black and proud and wearing it on our sleeves. I had an Afro hairstyle that rivaled Angela

Davis's for volume—as my husband likes to joke, it was so full that I had to walk sideways to get through a doorway. Hoop earrings and dashikis were my fashion staples.

In 1964 the Civil Rights Act was passed requiring all schools in the United States to end racial segregation. As part of the movement to integrate schools, I was selected by my high school principal to be the first African American to integrate the women's dormitory at a university, located in the Northeastern region of the United States, that was segregated by custom, not by law. To honor my father's legacy, as someone who fought to integrate the United States Armed Forces, my family and I agreed. At that time the only other African American students in attendance at the university were the basketball team, and the son of a well-known civil rights icon, whose mother thought his attendance at the university would honor his father's legacy as well. He and I became good friends.

My welcome to the university was a summons from the Dean of Women to her office, where she informed me that interracial dating was prohibited and that if I did so, I would be expelled. When I protested to the President of the University, not because I was interested in interracial dating, but because I felt insulted by the threat and the presumption that I was, he emphatically affirmed that this was indeed the university's policy. I was dumbfounded by his response. His lack of empathy and support shocked me and left me feeling invisible, isolated, and alone. In spite of this incident, and the seemingly endless emotional slights I experienced that centered on race, I stayed the full four years until I graduated, because I was committed to honoring my father's legacy and to making a difference. No dates. No sorority. One friend. I was lonely.

I will never know what difference, if any, my attendance at that university made to other people, or if it paved the way for others to have a better experience than I had, but what I do know is this. Staying in that environment for four years took a toll. As I look back on those years, I realize now it was nothing short of a traumatic experience, and one that I would not invite anyone else to go through. By the time I graduated from college, I was pretty beat up emotionally. I needed to recover from what had been the daily onslaught of racial wounding I had experienced for four years. In addition, now that I was working, I needed respite from the ongoing, recurrent episodes of negative race-related events I faced in my work environment—what we would commonly now call racial microaggressions.

THE HEALING BALM

I don't know how I discovered it, but by some quirk of fate, I stumbled upon a yoga class being offered at the local art museum. There were no yoga studios then. My teacher, I later discovered, was regarded as one of Paramahansa Yogananda's (*Autobiography of a Yogi*) foremost disciples. I did not know it at the time, but I was introduced to yoga by the teachings of a master. I attended his weekly yoga class as well as the Sunday services he offered, where he would read Paramahansa Yogananda's lectures and then lead a meditation practice. Nothing could keep me from attending those classes, where I learned about and experienced the healing power of self-love, self-care, and self-realization. We were given *The Autobiography of a Yogi* (1946) to read and we were instructed to practice asana (postures) and pranayama (breath techniques) on our own in between the once-a-week classes. Because of this approach, of necessity I became grounded in a home practice without realizing how advanced that actually was. Yoga helped heal my body, my mind, and my heart over 50 years ago. I have been practicing it ever since.

In the late 1990s yoga studios began to proliferate in the city where I lived. That is when I began to attend yoga studio classes with great regularity. To join with other students and to be taught by some pretty outstanding teachers was fun and challenging too. Like many practitioners, I decided to take yoga teacher training to learn more about the practice. It was in teacher training that I was introduced to Restorative Yoga. What I loved most about the Restorative Yoga practice was that it was practiced in stillness and silence and gave me a chance to notice my own internal workings. As a psychologist, this was very important to me, as much of my work involves helping people live consciously by becoming aware of their inner thoughts and feelings, and how those impact one's life and the lives of those you encounter. Restorative Yoga gave me deeper access to my interior life and supported emotional balance too. I taught Restorative Yoga with that in mind, hoping it would do the same thing for my students. I eventually began to share the practice with my psychotherapy clients as a therapeutic intervention, to help ease the suffering of emotional distress they experienced. The practice seemed like a perfect way to support people in the process of healing emotional wounds, to support self-study, and to bring ease and calm into turbulent and contracted lives.

WHY YOGA?

The purpose of yoga is to alleviate pain and suffering and to minimize it in the future. Over time it began to dawn on me that Restorative Yoga had a great deal to offer when it came to easing the emotional pain and suffering brought on by ethnic and race-based stress and trauma. Handling difficult life situations with composure is an important skill to hone. Dealing with race and ethnicity skillfully is critically important in a multiracial, multiethnic, multicultural world. Yoga practices, particularly Restorative Yoga, have much to offer when it comes to dealing with highly charged emotional issues like race and ethnicity. When we practice Restorative Yoga, we are teaching our nervous system how to release contraction and to feel safe coming into deep states of rest that support repair, rejuvenation, and resilience. We are developing a nervous system with a buffer, while strengthening our psychological immune system. When we learn to experience our emotional pain and discomfort without contracting around it and reacting to it, and instead just let it move through us, our nervous system becomes regulated and we become emotionally regulated. This means our nervous system is in a state of homeostasis, or balance, allowing us to see with more clarity, and we become grounded in a sense of well-being. As this happens, our responses to ethnic and racial offenses become wiser, more functional, and more effective.

Restorative Yoga for Ethnic and Race-Based Stress and Trauma is a book that offers a race-informed therapeutic approach to yoga. Everyone has a cultural context and a racial and ethnic identity. The argument can be made that we all have experiences, sometimes painful ones, that arise out of our racial and ethnic background. This book invites everyone to consider the psychological and emotional impact of ethnic and race-based stress and trauma, and it offers ways that yoga as a therapeutic tool can contribute to recovering from the emotional wounds that result.

Race-based traumatic stress is trauma that is associated with experiences of racial events that are negative and emotionally painful. An event can be experienced as race-related based on the individual's perception that a racist act occurred. Symptoms include defensiveness, anxiety, depression, anger, low self-esteem, shame, and sometimes guilt. Racial stress is a cumulative experience that is often magnified by the lack of opportunity to recover before the next experience, causing it to become chronic.

While therapies have been developed to address other forms of stress and trauma, there are currently few adequate therapeutic structures in place to help those who need it the most to process their experiences of racial stress and trauma. Racially informed Restorative Yoga and meditation practices can help by offering opportunities to step away from repeated experiences of ethnic and race-based wounding, while building the necessary stamina and resilience to develop effective coping strategies.

Today, we live in a complex world of difference that, in a positive way, we would call diversity. We are members of a global community, different from each other yet connected, often segregated, but not separate. As aware members of the human family, we know that when something affects one of us, it affects us all. But because we tend to live insular and segregated lives, many times we see our own views as the totality of the human experience and fail to understand or appreciate another person's reality. As perceptions of difference harden into prejudices and bias, we are at risk of being wounded or of wounding others. In either case, the experience can lead to stress and trauma, and the physical, emotional, psychological, and spiritual impact of that experience.

Yoga utilized as a therapeutic strategy has an opportunity to address a need by including self-care practices that are relevant to ethnic and racial experiences of stress and trauma. These practices are not just asana-based but include the philosophical precepts and contemplative practices of yoga as well. Yoga is a pathway toward personal transformation. It is subversive. It is an inside-out job that changes you bit by bit, over time. It transforms you by increasing physical balance and flexibility, then mentally and emotionally by slowing your mind and calming your emotions; it helps you think more clearly and helps you trust your intuitive abilities; it offers guidelines that support humane behavior; it aids you in listening to yourself and to others at deep and subtle levels; and, most importantly, it strengthens resilience and your capacity for self-love and self-acceptance, and gives you the courage to be truthful and honest in a compassionate way, not only with others but with yourself as well.

Because the yoga community is becoming more ethnically and racially diverse, the conversation within and around yoga, particularly yoga therapy and trauma-informed yoga, needs to keep pace with the shifting demographics. Maintaining a culture of silence regarding ethnicity and race makes that impossible. This book breaks that silence, begins the conversation, and suggests practices that can lead to recovering from ethnic and race-based stress and trauma. It will point to a pathway that allows yoga teachers and therapists, regardless of race and ethnicity, to prepare themselves to offer the practice.

Restorative Yoga is an important self-care strategy that supports physical, psychological, emotional, and spiritual health. It is ideal for those times we feel depleted or overwhelmed, or are recovering from an illness or a physical or psychological injury. It offers physical revitalization and psychological renewal, and fortifies us spiritually. It can be a buffer against secondary trauma and trauma in general, including race-based traumatic stress and White fragility. It helps us self-regulate, restore resilience, and establish physical and emotional balance. As we heal our own wounds, we can be more effective in addressing the needs of our families, our students, clients, patients, and our communities.

To that end, this book is intended to be a self-study and instructional guide in how to utilize and teach Restorative Yoga as a self-care practice to alleviate the pain and suffering of ethnic and race-based stress and trauma. It will include what race-based traumatic stress injury (RBTSI) is, how it differs from post-traumatic stress disorder (PTSD), where and how it lands in the body, and what can trigger it. It will explain how Restorative Yoga and meditation can help buffer the nervous system, increase stamina and resilience, strengthen the psychological immune system, and expand the window of tolerance for non-reactive responses to stressful situations. We will take a look at cultural conditioning regarding issues associated with race and ethnicity, including the cultural blind spots that make this a difficult topic to approach. We will explore the importance of creating conscious communities of care and support, and we will discuss activism from a spiritual perspective. It will also include instructions, with illustrations, in how to teach and practice Restorative Yoga and meditation. Reflections and Discussion topics will be offered at the end of each chapter as additional tools you can use to enhance self-study.

Restorative Yoga for Ethnic and Race-Based Stress and Trauma is written to aid you in the process of uncovering, examining, and healing your own emotional wounds and to help you avoid wounding or re-wounding others.

CHAPTER 1: THE WOUNDS HEAL BUT THE SCARS HURT

The goal of this chapter is to highlight the ethnic and racial diversity that exists within the world of yoga, and to bring awareness to the existence of race-based stress and trauma within that world. It discusses the potential of yoga to alleviate the distress associated with this type of emotional injury. It underscores how a lack of awareness of this form of stress and trauma can, and often does, result in re-traumatizing, and describes the emotional and psychological nature its impact has, with examples: who is impacted, and how one's context and lived experience influence the experience of race-based stress and trauma. This chapter includes a discussion on the mindful use of language, and the importance of self-study as it pertains to one's own relationship to race and ethnicity. It explores what the science says about race-based stress and trauma, including the effects of intergenerational trauma and ancestral memory, and points out how racial wounding can occur on the individual, institutional, and cultural level.

CHAPTER 2: HEALING THE WOUNDS OF RACIAL DISTRESS

This chapter establishes an empirical foundation for what race-based stress is; what race-based trauma is; whom it affects; how it differs from post-traumatic stress disorder (PTSD) and in what ways it is similar; how re-wounding occurs; how Restorative Yoga helps and why this is important to address. It discusses the context within which race-based stress and trauma occur, and hypothesizes that people who suffer from the ongoing stress and trauma of racial wounding can benefit from a practice that helps rest the body, relax the mind, release tension, process emotion, and build resilience. To support this hypothesis it includes: Dr. James T. Carter's Race-Based Traumatic Stress Injury Model; cultural anthropologist Dr. Leith Mullings's and epidemiologist Dr. Sherman James's research that uncovered a behavioral style people engage in to overcome the psychosocial factors and barriers to equality that lead to negative health outcomes; the wisdom of Patanjali's Yoga Sutra; personal as well as professional observation, along with common sense. It discusses Restorative Yoga's relevance as a self-care strategy that supports health and well-being, and its potential as a therapeutic healing modality.

CHAPTER 3: THE HEALING POWER OF RELATIONSHIP

This chapter is about the healing power of social engagement and the role a regulated nervous system plays in supporting it. It describes how the nervous system functions as an internal safety monitor that is always scoping for danger or safety, and how we create a narrative to match the state of the nervous system's response. The repetition of the narrative in our mind can continue to trigger the stress response and maintain and reinforce dysregulation of the nervous system. When the nervous system is dysregulated or out of balance, due to unhealed trauma, it registers signals of danger based on past experience, not on present-day reality, and interferes with our ability to engage with others in an optimal way. The chapter offers a brief description of the autonomic and parasympathetic nervous system; an overview of the polyvagal theory as developed by Dr. Stephen Porges, including the hierarchy of the nervous system's function, neuroception, dysregulation, and co-regulation of the nervous system. It highlights Restorative Yoga's ability to regulate the response of the nervous system and bring it into balance to support health and well-being, and the role the yoga therapist, teacher, or practitioner plays in utilizing the social engagement system to aid in nervous system regulation.

CHAPTER 4: ARE YOU IN YOUR SKIN?

The pain of racial wounding lands viscerally in the body, impacting the emotions and the mind. It is not uncommon for people who have been repeatedly emotionally injured or traumatized to become frozen or numb to the painful bodily sensations that accompany racial wounding. In the extreme, they may even experience dissociation—detachment from the mind or body. The chapter includes: an examination of the koshas, the subtle energy bodies; an examination of the pain body; samskaras, those repetitive patterns of behavior that occur outside of conscious awareness; interoception, the internal sense of the state of the body; some physical and emotional manifestations of race-based stress and trauma; emotional regulation; emotional triggers; and our emotional sweet spot, where body, mind, heart, and soul are in harmony. The chapter explains how to identify where emotional injury lands in the body, and how to ease the physical discomfort as well as the psychological impact on individuals. It describes how to identify areas of relaxation and how that affects one's sense of well-being. It describes how Restorative Yoga and the contemplative practices of yoga help mitigate the negative impacts of race-based stress and trauma, by offering experiences of feeling relaxed and feeling safe in stillness, allowing you to observe and identify how safety and relaxation feel in the body.

CHAPTER 5: SHINE A LIGHT

This chapter explores cultural conditioning regarding issues associated with race and ethnicity, including the culture of silence that makes this a difficult topic to approach. It includes an examination of the shadow side of self. The aim of the chapter is to bring awareness to cultural paradigms that influence our perceptions regarding race and ethnicity, that help maintain the status quo, and to offer new ways of thinking that challenge it. We see through the lens of cultural conditioning and attach meaning to our conditioned responses. The chapter discusses the impacts of cultural conditioning including the cultural paradigms of silence and color blindness; the use of the terms 'White privilege' and 'people of color'; the demonization of difference; the mythology of individualism and meritocracy; the dynamics of dominant and subordinated groups; the importance of challenging the assumptions we make about race and ethnicity based on our conditioning, as well as how to detect blind spots, and how to identify and gain insight into implicit and explicit biases through an examination of the kleshas.

CHAPTER 6: COMMUNITIES OF CARE

This chapter deals with envisioning and creating caring communities by considering the Ubuntu philosophy, "I am because we are," and by utilizing the yamas and niyamas as guideposts for creating caring communities. We are hardwired to be in connection and to feel safe in the company of others we know and trust. When we feel socially disconnected or excluded, we feel emotional pain. This pain is just as real as the pain we feel when we have been physically injured. This chapter invites readers to open their hearts and minds to each other, to go beyond being tolerant or politically correct in relationship to others, and instead to make being in connection with one another a priority. It invites us to recognize the commonness of our humanity, and emphasizes reciprocity and interpersonal relationship as the container for building bridges toward understanding across racial and ethnic differences.

CHAPTER 7: SPIRITUAL ACTIVISM— YOGA FROM THE INSIDE OUT

This chapter addresses activism from a spiritual perspective. It is about the importance of doing one's own inner healing work from racial wounding as an ongoing process. It is not possible to be helpful to anyone else if one is not engaged in self-reflection and self-regulation, and open to feedback from others about one's own biases and blind spots. The purpose of this chapter is to learn to sit in the discomfort of not knowing what to do when doing something seems necessary. If you act from a place of guilt, or shame, anger, or fear, you cannot be helpful to a situation that seems to require action. It is okay not to know what to do. It is not okay to do something anyway.

Healing from racial wounding can be painful. But the pain of healing is temporary. In order to be helpful, professionals must be willing to face their own pain and suffering in order to hold the space for others to heal. This chapter will include: a discussion on what spiritual activism is and the role the gunas play; the three stages of spiritual development; the power of stillness in our spiritual evolution; and the relationship between activism and spirituality.

CHAPTER 8: YOGA ON THE MAT

This chapter describes Restorative Yoga and meditation, how to teach and how to practice both. It includes: Restorative Yoga for resilience; the use of breath; the importance of spinal health; illustrations and descriptions of restorative poses; recommendations for soul care; how to create a Restorative Yoga class including postures and sequencing; meditation; and Yoga Nidra.

REFERENCES

Blakemore, E. (2018) "How dolls helped win Brown v. Board of Education." *History*. Accessed on 11/13/2019 at www.history.com/news/brown-v-board-of-education-doll-experiment.

DiAngelo, R. (2011) "White fragility." *International Journal of Critical Pedagogy 3*, 3, 54–70.

Elliott, J. (2017[1970]) *The Eye of the Storm*. Accessed on 11/13/2019 at www.youtube.com/watch?v=6gi2T0ZdKVc.

Peters, W. (1985) *A Class Divided*. Accessed on 11/13/2019 at www.pbs.org/wgbh/frontline/film/class-divided.

UChicago Magazine (2010) "A conversation with Margaret Beale Spencer." *Dialogo: UChicago Magazine*. Accessed on 11/13/2019 at https://mag.uchicago.edu/law-policy-society/conversation-margaret-beale-spencer#.

Yogananda, P. (1946) *Autobiography of a Yogi*. New York, NY: The Philosophical Library.

Chapter 1

THE WOUNDS HEAL
BUT THE SCARS HURT

W E RETAIN a memory of our injuries whether they are physical or psychological, even after the injury has healed and scarred over. Where scar tissue has formed, we can, from time to time, be reminded of the hurt. This is especially true of our deepest emotional wounds. Writing on the topic of race-based stress and trauma is like that for me. It scares me some. Maybe it's because it brings up old wounds from my past that are healed but scarred over. Maybe it's because I'm afraid of encountering wounds that have yet to be healed. Racial wounding is painful, and approaching those wounds risks reopening them because race-based stress and trauma linger. But our emotional scars are the marks that tell a story of times when life really hurt us but did not break us. They are indicators of our great strength and resilience. We need not be afraid to approach them or to show them. True healing comes when you learn to face your wounds, not hide them. Yoga as a therapeutic healing modality has an important role to play in helping us face and heal our emotional wounds.

Science has proven time and time again that yoga and meditation can reduce stress and anxiety, but for a variety of reasons the very people who need these practices most are often excluded from the benefits. Many people feel uncomfortable entering yoga studios, because it is just one more place where they risk being invalidated, rendered invisible, or treated as other. You might find this surprising, but I have had some experiences in yoga spaces that were as shocking as they were hurtful. I will share three of them with you—examples of what can happen when yoga teachers, practitioners, and yoga therapists lack critical awareness of race and racism and the emotional injury that results, not because they are trying to inflict pain, but because they are unaware of the pain that resides within their own bodies and in the bodies of those directly impacted. It is important to be able to respond in ways that are beneficial when issues of race and ethnicity surface, which they often do. I share these events because each of them represents a teachable moment.

TEACHABLE MOMENTS

I was in a fast-paced, vinyasa-style yoga class and the hip-hop music the yoga teacher selected for her playlist included the "n" word in the lyrics. No one seemed to notice but me. Rather than having an outburst right then and there, yoga helped me pause first and then take a deep breath. I spent the rest of the class formulating what I would say about the experience once the class was over. At the end of the class, I shared what I heard and how it made me feel. The teacher insisted that she didn't hear the lyric, smiled apologetically, and said, "I'm sorry." The rest of the people in the class lowered their gaze and looked away. No one else responded or offered any support. Instead, as we were leaving the class, I overheard people whisper to each other how uncomfortable they felt about me sharing my experience, and then someone asked me, "Why did you have to say something to the teacher in front of the entire class?" "Because it happened in front of the entire class," I said. "It was a teachable moment."

There were other experiences in yoga spaces that were surprising and upsetting, but the next most memorable one was a few years later when a yoga teacher used the verbal prompt "ghetto booty." We were in downward-facing dog. Everyone in the class seemed to know what she meant. I had to look around to see what she was talking about. Each student lifted her hips higher and stuck out her rear end. I was just as shocked this time as I was hearing the "n-word" lyric, but this time I had the presence of mind to say without hesitation, "What do you mean by that?" The teacher said, "Get your hips higher." So I said, "Then why don't you just give us that instruction?" And she said, with a big smile on her face, "Oh, okay, if that works better for you." And then she gave the "ghetto booty" prompt three more times.

Rather than leaving the class or getting into an argument with her, I once again used the remainder of the class to think about what I would say after class, and how I would say it—another teachable moment, I thought.

When the class ended, I took the teacher aside and asked her what came to mind when she used the term "ghetto booty." She said, "Nothing really. It's just an expression." I asked her what she thought her students imagined when she used that prompt. "I don't know," she said, "I never asked, but they usually just laugh and then lift their hips." I explained that "ghetto booty" is a cartoonish characterization of Black women's bodies, and that in case she didn't know it, when used by a non-Black person it becomes a racialized trope that reinforces a negative stereotype. A few participants in the class whispered to me afterward, "I'm so glad you said something. I didn't know what to say."

I will share one final example of why it is important for yoga teachers and therapists to develop awareness of ethnic and race-based stress and trauma, and why it is important to learn effective tools that can adequately address the emotionally charged issues of race and ethnicity when they come up in yoga spaces. I attended a workshop describing the benefits of yoga for elementary school students. During the question-and-answer period, someone stated that she had just begun teaching yoga in an inner-city school and that all of her students were "of color." She wondered how, given the difference in socioeconomic status, race, and ability between her and her students, she could best relate to them. You could feel the tension in the room. There was an extended period of silence in response to her question. It was clear that people were triggered because no one in the room seemed to know how to respond, and no one seemed to be breathing. It was a painfully awkward moment for the workshop presenters and for those of us in attendance, including the woman who asked the question.

In circumstances like this when we are triggered emotionally, in order to make ourselves and others feel better, it is tempting to manage the discomfort by ignoring it altogether, or by becoming confrontational as a way of correcting or challenging the person who triggered the discomfort. The problem is, avoidance ignores the situation and changes nothing, and confrontation shuts down communication, minimizes opportunities for deeper intrapersonal and interpersonal growth and understanding, and can make matters worse. Unless and until we deal with our own discomfort regarding issues of race and ethnicity, and unless we learn the necessary tools to address emotional discomfort in a constructive, non-defensive, non-confrontational, non-avoidant way, opportunities for deeper understanding and connection are missed.

Yoga offers us a starting point. The breath. In the instance I just described, it was clear by the extended silence, and the fact no one seemed to be exhaling, that people were triggered by the question. So we start by reminding people to breathe. Reminding people to breathe in an emotionally uncomfortable situation is no different from the instruction yoga teachers and therapists use all the time when you notice that no one is breathing in physical postures. Remember, yoga is a breath practice. Breathing encourages relaxation and calm, and helps focus your awareness internally. It gives you time to pause before you react out of a sense of your own discomfort, which is never a good time to respond. Trying to respond to an emotionally charged situation before addressing your own internal discomfort puts the cart before the horse.

Next, instead of trying to answer a triggering question or criticizing it, invite the person to explore the answer to her own question. By doing this you are helping the questioner cultivate an internal focus. You might respond by inviting the person, "Tell us what you know about the answer to your question." This intervention invites an internal focus and puts the onus and responsibility for the answer onto the questioner where it belongs. It avoids shaming, blaming, or criticizing, and takes the focus off of how you might answer her question. It gives the person a chance to hear herself and empowers her to realize that she may know more than she realizes about the answer to her own question. Additionally, it teaches those in attendance how to manage discomfort in a way that supports self-reflection.

Contemplating what you know about the answer to the questions you ask requires self-reflection and awareness, and requires you to dig deep within yourself for answers. When you do this, your question becomes a tool of self-study. No one can teach you what your relationship to race and ethnicity is, or even tell you what it should be, nor can you teach anyone else. But once you have learned how to access your inner world and gain insight into your own thoughts, feelings, attitudes, and beliefs, you can teach that to others. Shining a light on your thoughts, attitudes, and beliefs about race and ethnicity, the ones you may have previously ignored, is how real change begins. Remember, this is an inside-out job. This is about change through personal transformation. This is about self-study.

We live in a culture that is complicit in its silence about racial issues. Because of this silence, many of us are ignorant about our inner relationship to ethnicity and race. I speak up, not because I necessarily want to, and certainly not because it's easy or safe. I speak up, when I do, because I understand that silence can be corrosive and, in some cases, though not all, even more dangerous than speaking up. The thoughts we think and the language we use matter. Words have power to hurt or to heal. How many of you remember hearing "Sticks and stones may break my bones, but words will never hurt me"? It's not true. Words may not break bones, but they can break hearts. There are words that hurt far worse than any physical blow that could be levied. There are words and practices, however, that heal, nourish the soul, strengthen, inspire, and help you bounce back. Our work, regardless of one's race or ethnicity, is to use words that heal and support growth.

When you approach speaking as a part of your yoga practice, you become conscious of the language you use and how it impacts other people. When you practice speaking following the principle of non-harming, ahimsa in Sanskrit, you choose words carefully that communicate reverence and respect. Working with mantra, which is the repetition of a sacred sound such as Om, or words like "love" or "peace," can help shift your speech patterns by recalibrating the energy in your physical and subtle bodies, creating an internal environment that gives your words new clarity and power.

Yoga as a sacred practice requires the use of reverent and respectful language. As yogis, practitioners, teachers, and therapists, we have a responsibility to be mindful of our thoughts and to use language in a respectful, conscious, instructive, and constructive way. We are teaching and affecting others. It is never enough just to know what you are teaching, although that is essential. But equally important is taking into consideration what people are learning, and how they are being affected by what you are teaching. Before you speak, it is important to ask yourself, "What impact do I want to have?" "What impact am I having?" "Does the impact I want to have match the impact I am having?" And finally, "What is the outcome I am trying to create?"

WHO PRACTICES YOGA?

An internet search shows estimates of the number of yoga practitioners worldwide ranging between two billion (UN News 2016) and 200 to 300 million people (The Good Body 2016). According to a study commissioned by *Yoga Journal* and Yoga Alliance (Yoga Journal 2016), 36.7 million

Americans are practicing yoga. The study included what it called the general population, defined as all Americans including practitioners, teachers, and studio owners. It tracked the respondents' age, gender, and region of the country, but did not include income, ethnic, or racial demographics as part of the study. The *Journal of Behavioral Medicine* (Park, Braun, and Siegel 2015) reported that the practice of yoga in the United States has been consistently dominated by a White racial group demographic. The research showed that African Americans, Asian Americans, Latinex, Native Americans, Asian Pacific Islanders, and Native Alaskans are a significant minority of all Americans practicing yoga. It also indicated that 48 percent of yoga practitioners earned a household income of at least $65,000 per year. All you have to do is attend a public yoga class almost anywhere in the United States to recognize that the majority of yoga practitioners and teachers fit the dominant racial group demographic, and the stereotype of the thin, middle- to upper-class, 30–49-year-old female yogi cited in this study. Given this, it is easy to see how the values, beliefs, and historical perspectives, whether consciously or unconsciously, can be culturally imposed on people who have different values, beliefs, and experiences based on race, ethnicity, religion, nationality, gender, age, body size, sexual orientation, and socioeconomic status.

People of all races, ethnicities, and cultures have always practiced yoga, as can be seen in the video *The Uncommon Yogi: A History of Blacks and Yoga in the U.S.* (Long 2016), and have embraced yoga practices as a wellness strategy to take care of themselves, de-stress, and heal. More people of various races and ethnicities are teaching yoga too. As the yoga community becomes more racially and ethnically diverse, it is incumbent upon yoga teachers and yoga therapists to become aware of the existence of racial stress and trauma, and to address this directly so that we are not guilty of causing harm through neglect, or by attitudes, actions, or the language we use. It is safe to assume that any person of color walking through the door of a yoga studio or entering into a therapeutic relationship has experienced some form of race-based stress or trauma, whether they acknowledge it or not. It is unlikely that they are practicing yoga or coming to yoga therapy for the purpose of addressing it directly, but that does not mean that the pain of racial or ethnic wounding does not surface or get triggered in yoga spaces. It inevitably will for a variety of reasons. There is a need in the yoga community to delve into yoga as a healing balm for race-based stress and trauma so that yoga can benefit everyone.

Yoga communities in the United States are a microcosm of the macrocosm. As the country becomes more racially and ethnically diverse, so do yoga communities. Because of this the conversation within and around yoga needs to expand to keep pace with the shifting demographics. Yoga is a holistic practice. It means union, the connection of body, mind, and heart, the connection of breath to movement, the connection of one human being to another. It is an invitation to intimacy with oneself and connection to others—even to those who are different from us. Disconnections are caused by behaviors and language that make a person feel odd, invisible, like an outsider, and unwelcome. Connections are strengthened when conversations take place that make a person feel respected and understood. This requires curiosity, cultural awareness, cultural humility, cultural competence, and a willingness to have open, non-defensive conversations. It means opening your heart to others who are different from you and offering your perspective as well as listening to theirs. It means a willingness to engage with them and to be changed by your engagement with them. That is yoga.

ETHNIC AND RACE-BASED STRESS AND TRAUMA

"This may sound like a stupid question, but I'll ask it anyway. In what way is race-based stress different from other forms of stress? I mean physiologically is there any difference?" A woman from Denmark asked this question regarding a workshop I was conducting on Restorative Yoga for race-based stress and trauma. I didn't think it was a stupid question at all. I actually thought it was a pretty good one. I explained that what makes race-based stress and trauma unique is not the physiology but the context in which it occurs and the psychological and emotional impact it has. All of us live within a historical, cultural, racial, and ethnic context. Whether we are aware of it or not, we each have stories to tell, some more painful than others, about experiences that we have had that have shaped our consciousness regarding our racial and ethnic identity. This is why it is important for us to understand context.

In the United States, news reports abound with stories describing race-related events that target non-Whites. In 2018 two young men were arrested in a coffee shop for trespassing while they waited for a business associate to arrive. When they declined to order anything while they waited, the store manager called the police. The police arrived, handcuffed them, took them into custody, and held them for nine hours before releasing them. Even though they were treated like criminals, they were not charged with a crime because they had not committed one. In another incident one month later, police escorted a female graduate student attending an Ivy League University out of a common area where she fell asleep studying, after a fellow student called police saying she didn't think the woman looked as if she belonged there. The student had to show her identification to the police to prove that in fact she was enrolled in the university. Later that same year, when the referee of a high school wrestling match demanded it, rather than being allowed to use his headgear to cover his hair before the match, a student wrestler suffered the public humiliation of having his dreadlocks cut off by the trainer of his high school wrestling team, under threat of forfeiting his high school team's match if he didn't permit it.

What each of these individuals, who were confronted by authorities, had in common was race and ethnicity. They were Black. What the people who reported them to authorities had in common was race. They were White, as were the authority figures. These events are painful reminders of how vulnerable black and brown bodies can be in predominantly White spaces. I could not have anticipated or predicted the experiences of racial insensitivity that occurred in the yoga spaces I described. I am sure that not placing an order while waiting for someone you are meeting in a coffee shop, falling asleep in a common study area at the university you pay to attend, and wearing dreadlocks to your wrestling match, as you had done many times before with no penalty, are not behaviors that anyone could have anticipated would attract the kind of aggressive and hostile response these young people received.

THE BLIND MAN AND THE ELEPHANT

Each of us creates a unique view of the world based on our limited experience of it. A common mistake is to assume that what we see and experience is the whole truth. There is an ancient Indian parable called "The Blind Man and the Elephant" that illustrates how limiting this can be.

Once upon a time, there were six blind sages living in the same village. They had never seen an elephant but had always wanted to. One day an elephant came to the village and they finally had their chance. They asked a guide to lead them to the elephant. When they arrived each of the men used his hands as his eyes by touching the elephant to determine what it was like. The first sage touched the elephant's side and concluded that the elephant was like a wall. The second sage touched the elephant's leg and concluded that the elephant was like a tree trunk. The third sage touched the elephant's ear and concluded that the elephant was like a fan. The fourth sage touched the elephant's trunk and concluded that the elephant was like a fat snake. The fifth sage touched the elephant's tusk and concluded that the elephant was like a spear. The sixth sage touched the elephant's tail and concluded that the elephant was like a rope. Not realizing that he had only touched a part of the elephant, each sage assumed that the part he touched was the entire elephant. Based on that assumption, they each determined what the elephant looked like. They argued endlessly trying to convince each other that their version of the elephant was the right version.

The parable illustrates that seeing from your own perspective, as if yours is the only one, blinds you to the bigger picture and to the perspective of others. Each of us is perceiving reality through our own unique lens, influenced by our beliefs, values, race, ethnicity, culture, and life experiences. We are not all seeing and responding to the same thing.

We filter information through our own lived experience and take in what we can from our own perspective. An event is regarded as race-related when the person experiencing it perceives it that way. It is subjective. Yoga teaches us to honor our own and others' lived experience. If you are not living the experience of racial wounding, the events I have described may be hard to believe and may seem unusual and unlikely, but that does not mean they are nonexistent. If you are living the experience, you know that these events are not uncommon. So how do people living the experience daily describe it? I took an informal poll to find out.

GOOD MORNING STRESS

An African American physician calls it death by a thousand cuts, the daily emotional assaults that take a toll physiologically, psychologically, and spiritually. He says for him it begins first thing in the morning. On his drive to work he is constantly worried about being pulled over by police. He goes through the same thing on his way home from work every day. Once he is at work, he crosses every "T" and dots every "I." Zero tolerance for error is the standard he sets for himself. It is an incredibly stressful one, he admits, but one he feels he must adhere to for his professional survival because, based on experience, he cannot assume he will be given the benefit of the doubt. He says he never feels fully relaxed at mixed-race social gatherings, because he is on guard for an unexpected racially charged remark. He is wary of going into unfamiliar places because he can never be certain of how he will be perceived or received; will he be refused service, ignored, dismissed, or followed around by someone suspicious that he may be up to no good? Will someone call the police? He never knows. He doesn't let any of this stop him, but he never feels as if he can let down his guard. On top of all of that, he says he is fearful each and every day for the safety of his wife and son.

A nine-year-old boy who lives in a racially mixed community with his mother tells her after visiting his father, who lives in a predominantly White suburb, "White people smile with their mouths but not with their eyes. When they see me and Daddy, they stare, and the White ladies always hug their purse or walk across the street when they see us coming." His mother says it breaks her heart to know that her son is having this experience, and she wonders what it is like for him to walk around with his father and be perceived as a threat. She wonders how it will be for him when he is independent enough to walk through the world on his own. She is fearful for him and wonders how to raise him not to be afraid when she herself is terrified for his safety. She worries about how to help him build his self-confidence going forward.

An Indian American woman, born and raised in the United States by immigrant parents, says she feels fearful daily because she knows that she is perceived as an immigrant. Growing up, she saw how her parents were mistreated because of their immigrant status and brown skin. She worries about her own and her children's safety because even though they were all born in the United States, they receive second-class treatment because of their "foreign" appearance. She wonders if she did the right thing by giving her children Indian first names and feels ashamed that she even wonders that. Her mother, a naturalized citizen, is reluctant to take her grandchildren across the Canadian border to see Niagara Falls, for fear of being treated disrespectfully by border guards when she tries to re-enter the United States. She doesn't want to risk exposing her grandchildren to observing any abusive behavior that she might be subjected to.

On top of these daily stressors, each of these people describes reliving traumatic events from the past while they accumulate new experiences every day. Human beings are resilient and adapt to their circumstances. Managing fear, pain, and anguish is a necessary form of survival in a culture that is afraid of or hostile toward you, has rules and customs that do not always apply to you, and that discriminates against and alienates you. The ability to navigate safety when you know you are perceived as a threat is an important skill to learn, but learning that skill alone does not heal the pain. Even worse, it masks it, and there is a cost to one's physical and emotional health and well-being.

Now imagine that one or all three of the people I polled about their lived experience of race-based stress come to a yoga class—and, by the way, they all do practice yoga—or come to you for yoga therapy. It is unlikely that they are coming to your class or to therapy for the express purpose of sharing the stresses I have described, so you would never know any of these details. But what you should know is that they are bringing their history of ethnic and racial stress and trauma, and their coping behaviors into the space with them. If part of your history includes being treated with suspicion, being treated as insignificant, or being treated as less than, and you arrive at a yoga studio in your yoga outfit with your yoga mat in tow 15 minutes before class, and are greeted with "Oh, are you here for yoga?," how would you feel? How would you interpret that? If you enter a crowded yoga room and no one moves to make room for you, and no one does anything to facilitate that, how do you think that would make you feel? How would you interpret that? When the yoga teacher asks people in the class to pair off to do a partnered asana, and you are the only person in the room left without a partner, and no one facilitates that, how do you think that would make you feel? How would you interpret that? Do you think you would return?

Each of the experiences I have described is an experience that has actually occurred, and there are untold numbers of stories like these. If you don't believe me, all you have to do is ask. Why do you suppose this is happening? Is everyone being treated with the same recognition, respect, and regard? If not, why not? Yoga classes and therapeutic yoga do not have to focus on race-based stress and trauma to be helpful. When the yoga teacher or yoga therapist has an awareness of the impacts of ethnic and race-based stress and trauma, and recognizes the potential of yoga practices to support the necessary strengths and resilience of those having the daily lived experience, that awareness, in and of itself, can be healing.

When I first began practicing yoga in studios, whenever a teacher would touch my head and massage my neck during savasana, I would have an instant tension reflex and recall all the times people had made demeaning remarks about my hair. I would freeze. Even though I knew the teacher's touches were loving or certainly neutral, and that she had no idea of my history, her touches brought up emotionally painful memories of negative comments made by others about my texturized hair, going all the way back to childhood. These were not memories I ever shared with my teachers, but they surfaced. Yoga taught me to just rest in the observation of the experience, and over time I was able to receive the touch without being triggered by it. Gradually, the practice of resting in my discomfort with awareness shifted from uncomfortable flashbacks into a simple curiosity about how my hair felt to the teacher when she touched it. I never asked. These experiences taught me that as yoga teachers and therapists we need to be sensitive to those in the room, and to what we do not know about them, and to be informed about and sensitive to the nuances of race-based stress. Without that awareness, the hidden stress and trauma of those living in racially oblivious or racially hostile environments can easily be exacerbated and re-traumatizing can occur.

INTERGENERATIONAL AND ANCESTRAL MEMORY

Ethnic and racial stress and trauma carry both physiological and psychological effects, leaving scars for those who are dehumanized by its impact. Some of the effects include being on high alert to threat; nightmares; aversion to certain people or experiences; flashbacks; headaches; stomach disorders; rapid heartbeat; insomnia; anxiety and depression, to name a few. Additionally, the cumulative experiences of racial stress and trauma over generations, caused by the historical trauma of genocide, enslavement, colonization, and dislocation, left unaddressed and unhealed, have intergenerational impact. Yes, the effects of racial stress and trauma go beyond the individuals who are directly impacted and affect entire communities for generations to come.

Dr. Joy DeGruy, a renowned researcher and social work professional, describes in her book *Post Traumatic Slave Syndrome* (DeGruy 2005) how present-day life experiences, reactions, attitudes, and behaviors of African

Americans to external events of racial trauma and stress are associated with the historical traumatic experiences of their enslaved ancestors. She describes how slavery produced centuries of physical, psychological, and emotional injury even after the fact. Her work was groundbreaking as she described attitudes, behaviors, and reactions passed down from one generation to the next, associated with intergenerational race-based stress and trauma.

As it turns out, people of all races, ethnicities, and cultures are impacted by intergenerational trauma. Resmaa Menakem, a psychotherapist and trauma specialist, addresses the unhealed intergenerational trauma of people in his book *My Grandmother's Hands* (Menakem 2017). He weaves together race, trauma, and biology, and states that racial attitudes are not just conceptual but are deep-seated bodily responses to unhealed trauma. He describes the trauma that Europeans endured during the Middle Ages when powerful white bodies tortured less powerful white bodies for hundreds of years. He traces how the trauma of these experiences was embedded in the white body and passed down from one generation to the next. One of the results, he says, manifests in what he refers to as "white body-supremacy," a response to unhealed intergenerational and historical trauma that elevates white bodies over others. He suggests that white ethnic and racial xenophobia, insensitivity, cruelty, oblivion, indifference, and harm are caused by unhealed traumatic retention.

Ancestral memory is real and makes a lasting imprint. We understand that genetic inheritance influences how we look: eye color, body structure, hair texture and skin color, illnesses we may be predisposed to, as well as our longevity. All of this exists outside of conscious awareness. But whether you know it or not, ancestral memory also resides in our attitudes, beliefs, and behaviors. We first learn about the world by interacting with and observing family members, all of whom first learned about the world from their ancestors, traumatic retentions and all. Ancestral memory influences your interpretation of life, your preferences, how you get your basic needs met, your perceptions of reality, how you achieve your goals, whom you love, how you love, whom you choose to be around, as well as ethnic and racial bias. Because ancestral memory tends to operate beneath conscious awareness, unless we become conscious of and recognize the traumatic patterns that originated in the history of our ancestors, we will more than likely bring them into our own lives, repeat them, and pass them on. This is true regardless of your racial identity.

The scientific understanding of emotional injury caused by racism is increasing. Behavioral science is catching up to the impact of daily lived experiences of ethnic and racial oppression, insensitivity, injustice, discrimination, and violence that affect a person's mental, physical, and emotional health and well-being. The entire first edition of the 2019 *American Psychologist* is entitled "Racial Trauma: Theory, Research, and Healing" (Comas-Díaz, Hall, and Neville 2019). The research included in the journal shows that people are stressed and traumatized by individual, institutional, and cultural occurrences of racism. The fact that scientific research on racial and ethnic injury is growing is good, but the human beings that suffer from race-based stress and trauma need solutions for healing the wounding caused by race-related events of ignorance, discrimination, harassment, injustice, and violence, more than they need another scientific study to describe what they are already experiencing. While we are waiting for the science to catch up, the greater need now is for self-care practices designed to ease the distress imposed by living in and navigating within a racialized culture.

REFLECTION

Therapeutic Journal Writing

When it comes to healing emotional wounds regarding race and ethnicity, it is important that we have opportunities to share our experiences so we can digest and process what happened. Sharing our stories supports resilience. Keeping our experiences to ourselves, which is frequently the case when stressful or traumatic events occur, is not healthy. When we are unable to process what happened, the trauma or stress-related injury does not heal; it is just pushed outside of awareness and remains stuck in our memory bank and in our bodies. Carrying around unprocessed feelings can be toxic, costing you peace of mind, happiness, and even your health.

When we shine a light on the hidden places within ourselves that are wounded, we can safely avoid their stress-related consequences. If you are fortunate enough to have someone you trust who can be a compassionate, empathic listener, not someone who feels sorry for you, wants to fix you, or make you feel better, or who becomes outraged and offended along with you, by all means open up to that person. But remember, there is a difference between expressing your feelings with someone for the purpose of processing a stressful or traumatic event and airing your grievance by going on a rant. Airing your grievance focuses more on your dissatisfaction or outrage about the event than on the feelings evoked by the event. To that end, healing is delayed because the focus is external, not internal. Sharing yourself for the purpose of processing stress or trauma involves expressing yourself with self-reflective awareness, focusing more on how you were emotionally impacted, and what you felt, than on the event itself.

If you do not have someone you trust with whom you can share your painful experiences, or you are just not ready to be that vulnerable, you can journal. The simple act of expressing your thoughts and emotions on paper about stressful and traumatic events can help you process and digest the feelings you experienced. Journal writing gives you an opportunity to deepen your understanding of your responses to the events of racial wounding that you have experienced, and helps you realize that even though you were victimized, you are not a victim. It is empowering, can bring clarity, and enable you to place your experience within the context of a larger narrative: your history, your intergenerational trauma, your ancestral memory, your strengths, your resilience, and your options for any action you need to take. It helps you realize that the stress or trauma you experienced is not your fault.

The Healing Power of Journal Writing

Therapeutic journal writing is one way to approach addressing the wounds of ethnic and race-related stress and trauma. Psychologist James Pennebaker discovered in his research that writing about emotionally upsetting events can result in better physical and psychological health. In his paradigm, the focus of therapeutic journal writing pays more attention to the feelings you experienced at the time of the event than the event itself.

The Pennebaker Paradigm (Pennebaker 2004) involves writing in a journal about a traumatic event, non-stop, without editing or censoring yourself, for 15–20 minutes at a time, for four days in a row. It involves writing about how you felt and why you felt the way you did at the time of the event. Each day you are instructed to add on layers as you write, including facts and feelings about what happened, how you were impacted, how it has influenced you, and how you feel about the event once you have explored it in writing.

DISCUSSION

- What is your racial group identity?
- When and how did you discover you had a racial identity?
- Have you ever been treated as if you were inferior because of your race or ethnicity?
- Have you ever been given preferential treatment because of your race or ethnicity?
- What is your first memory of racial or ethnic wounding?
- What is your first memory of hurting someone of another race or ethnicity?
- Are you aware of any trauma in your family's history?
- How do you think you have been impacted?

REFERENCES

Comas-Díaz, L., Hall, G.N., and Neville, H.A. (2019) "Racial trauma: Theory, research, and healing: Introduction to the special issue." *American Psychologist* 74, 1, 1–5.

DeGruy, J. (2005) *Post Traumatic Slave Syndrome.* Portland, OR: Joy DeGruy Publications.

Long, J. (2016) *The Uncommon Yogi: A History of Blacks and Yoga in the U.S.* Accessed on 11/15/2019 at www.youtube.com/watch?v=xQqSdB9PD38.

Menakem, R. (2017) *My Grandmother's Hands.* Las Vegas, NV: Central Recovery Press.

Park, C.L., Braun, T., and Siegel, T. (2015) "Who practices yoga? A systematic review of demographic, health-related, and psychosocial factors associated with yoga practice." *Journal of Behavioral Medicine* 38, 3, 460–471.

Pennebaker, J.W. (2004) *Writing to Heal: A Guided Journal for Recovering from Trauma and Emotional Upheaval.* Oakland, CA: New Harbinger Publications.

The Good Body (2018) "Yoga statistics: Staggering growth shows ever increasing popularity." Accessed on 11/13/2019 at www.thegoodbody.com/yoga-statistics.

UN News (2016) "Two billion people practice yoga 'because it works.'" Accessed on 11/13/2019 at https://news.un.org/en/audio/2016/06614172.

Yoga Journal (2016) "2016 Yoga in America Study conducted by Yoga Journal and Yoga Alliance." Accessed on 11/13/2019 at www.yogajournal.com/page/yogainamericastudy.

Chapter 2

HEALING THE WOUNDS OF RACIAL DISTRESS

IN ORDER for therapeutic interventions to have validity, there need to be empirically, theoretically, philosophically, and culturally informed frameworks that support the intervention. From a psychological perspective, the Race-Based Traumatic Stress Injury Model will serve as a conceptual guide that supports a self-care strategy that has the potential to ease the distress caused by events of ethnic and racial wounding. From a yogic perspective, the Yoga Sutra of Patanjali will guide the way. From a culturally informed perspective, high-effort coping will be presented as a behavioral style, used to combat and overcome psychosocial barriers to success and equal opportunity that can compromise physical and emotional health. Lived experiences and culturally informed studies and perspectives will also be offered.

The Race-Based Traumatic Stress Injury Model is a model that focuses on the harm caused by race-related events, not on fixing the reaction of the person who has been harmed (Carter 2007). It holds the view that race-related events that cause stress and trauma are forms of emotional injury, and that the various emotional responses that people exhibit are not pathological in nature. Understood within the context of the person's racial and/or ethnic identity, culture, history, and lived experience, their reactions are regarded as adaptive responses to emotional pain.

Pathologizing responses to the emotional harm caused by race-related events, as if the response is the problem, actually invalidates the experience of racial wounding and is in and of itself harmful. It places the responsibility for the wound on the one who is wounded, and not on the event or the one who causes the wound. I am always deeply touched by the relief people express when I tell them that their responses to the hurt and suffering they experience, caused by race-related events, make sense and do not mean that there is something wrong with them. Knowing that your responses to pain and suffering are normal responses to being hurt, and not an indication that there is something wrong with you, is empowering. This does not mean that emotional pain and suffering should be ignored. Pain serves an important protective function. It triggers a reflexive response signaling us to withdraw from something harmful. Just as you would attend to a physical wound to help it heal, your emotional wounds need to be attended to as well. If you do not do the healing work necessary, your unhealed wounds can fester, worsen, and become deeply problematic.

Carter's research shows that race-related events are not only stressful but are traumatic too. He identifies race-based traumatic stress injury as any perceived race-related stress or trauma that is triggered by an external event that is memorable, comes as a surprise, is outside of your control, and causes emotional pain (Carter 2007). His research identifies three categories of racial injury that people are exposed to: discriminatory practices, such as being ignored or refused service in a store, or being denied housing or a bank loan; hostile forms of harassment, such as police profiling, being followed around in a store as if you are about to commit a crime, name calling, physical threats, and stereotyping; and finally the most subtle and potentially damaging form, discriminatory harassment, such as being denied a promotion at work, having your credentials or qualifications labeled as insufficient or invalid, or not being given the benefit of the doubt in various situations, and then being told that none of this has anything to do with race (Carter *et al.* 2016). The ambiguous nature of discriminatory harassment is the most damaging because it leaves the target unable to determine whether or not they did something wrong, leading to unwarranted self-blame. More dangerously, it undermines one's confidence in the ability to trust reality as it is experienced. It is a form of racial gaslighting.

Ethnic and race-based traumatic stress injury are ongoing, recurrent, and cumulative, and not something you get over easily or quickly, because in a racialized world events of ethnic and race-based stress and trauma are likely to occur anytime, anywhere, and without warning over a lifetime.

EMOTIONAL HARM

There is a video posted on social media that went viral. You may have seen it. It shows two young men being arrested in a coffee shop for trespassing because they declined to place an order while they waited for a business associate to arrive for a pre-arranged meeting. The store manager called the police with no apparent provocation, and without warning the young men that she would do so. Even though this coffee shop is well known for being a gathering place for customers to engage in conversation, have business meetings, work on their computers, and to just hang out, these two men were stereotyped as criminals, a common and dangerous stereotype projected onto African American men, and they were treated accordingly. When the police arrived, the young men were handcuffed, arrested, and held in custody for nine hours before being released. They had not committed a crime. Witnesses to the event said they were perplexed because they sit in this particular coffee shop all the time without ordering anything and have never been asked to leave, and no one has ever called the police. The only difference they could see between the ones being arrested and the ones who were not was race.

For the purposes of this discussion, what is important about the video I just described is the look of stoicism on the faces of the young men as they are being walked out of the coffee shop in handcuffs. In the video they are silent, showing no resistance to being arrested, and showing no emotion whatsoever. Now, put yourself in their position. How do you imagine you would feel under the circumstances? My guess is that you would be feeling some kind of way, and my guess is that even though they are showing no emotion, these young men were feeling some kind of way, but of necessity held their feelings in check. In a television interview following the event, even though they did not say so, it is clear by the look on their faces that they were still experiencing the hurt and humiliation that the incident caused. We hold stress and trauma in the body.

Race-based stress and trauma cause emotional distress and have a lasting impact. There are a range of responses to being discriminated against including fear, tension, anxiety, depression, sadness, anger, low self-esteem, suspiciousness, distrust, shame, and guilt. Carter's research shows that discriminatory racial encounters result in reactions of hyper-vigilance and arousal. He found that harassment-based race-related events are more closely associated with depression and other forms of emotional distress, and that events of harassment seem to have longer-lasting impact than events of discrimination (Carter *et al.* 2013). But he also found that the intention to overcome barriers to equal treatment, and the determination to use encounters of discrimination and harassment as sources of personal and community strength, are also responses to ethnic and race-related events (Carter 2007). In a televised interview, the young men who were arrested at the coffee shop, even though visibly shaken by the situation, said that they were committed to using the event to be an inspiration for others to persevere in the face of the kind of harassment and discrimination they will likely face in their lives.

SOCIAL EXCLUSION

One of the most emotionally painful experiences a human being faces is social exclusion. As it turns out, whether it is discrimination-based, harassment-based, or a combination of discrimination and harassment, ethnic and race-based social exclusion can be just as painful as a broken leg, a blinding headache, or a cramped stomach. Pain researchers have discovered that the reason social exclusion is so painful is that social and physical pain actually share the same neural pathway; they overlap (Eisenberger 2012). In other words, social pain registers in the body and it really does hurt physically. You're not making it up. When you ignore or minimize emotional pain, you do so to your detriment.

As children, we learn to hide our feelings, especially feelings of vulnerability, making it difficult to detect our emotional injuries. Over time we can lose the ability to even know when we are hurt. Racial wounding is like that. It is so common that it becomes normalized, ultimately minimized, and eventually denied. When you lose the ability to recognize it for what it is, abusive and traumatizing, and learn to tolerate the intolerable, the unacknowledged pain does not disappear; it just goes underground and can express itself in self-defeating, self-sabotaging behaviors that sap your vitality and make it difficult to live your best life. Procrastination, self-medicating with drugs or alcohol, emotional eating, spending money you do not have on things you do not need are a few examples.

Just as traumatizing as being a direct target of ethnic and racial hostility and discrimination is witnessing events of racial harm. The trauma of secondary exposure to a racially charged event is the experience of helplessness and fear that comes from seeing something that is emotionally overpowering. Imagine how you might feel if your son, daughter, husband, wife, sibling, child, friend, co-worker, or community member had been one of the people arrested in the coffee-shop incident. Imagine how you would be impacted in the event of exposure to a physically violent incident you might witness that involved someone you know or identify with. Imagine the impact of witnessing these events over and over again, in news reports, on social media, or even in your work life. The effects are pernicious.

POST-TRAUMATIC STRESS DISORDER

Claims of post-traumatic stress disorder (PTSD) have become part of popular parlance and are not necessarily based on a clinical diagnosis. It is not uncommon to hear people declare, when they are stressed out, that they suffer from PTSD. As a clinician, I have no doubt that many of us do suffer from both diagnosed and undiagnosed PTSD. I believe we are a society embedded in a state of unhealed cumulative trauma. Just think about the aftermath of war alone, and the visible and invisible effects that trauma has on soldiers, their families, friends, acquaintances, and entire communities, not to mention the traumatized people actually living in and fleeing from war zones. I grew up in the military and I am old enough to have experienced, as a young child, the trauma of the Korean War, as an adolescent and young adult, the trauma of the Vietnam War, and as a mature adult, the secondary trauma brought on by wars in the Middle East. As a society, we are unaware of our unresolved trauma and its effects, including the effects of the unhealed wounds of ethnic and race-based stress and trauma. We are traumatized physiologically and emotionally.

Post-traumatic stress disorder (PTSD) is regarded as a mental health disorder that is triggered by a life-threatening event that leaves the individual unable to shake off the trauma. Symptoms include unwanted intrusive thoughts, avoidance, hyper-vigilance/reactivity, low self-esteem, negative emotional states, and risky behaviors. These symptoms may lessen but can remain even after treatment.

Race-based traumatic stress injury (RBTSI) is not the same as post-traumatic stress disorder and should not be confused with it or treated in the same way. Even though the symptoms are similar to the symptoms associated with PTSD, the RBTSI model takes a different approach to stress and trauma. What distinguishes it from PTSD is the core stressor of the trauma. Race-based traumatic stress injury is triggered by emotionally painful race-related events rather than a threat to one's life (Carter *et al.* 2017).

Frequent exposure to race-related events intensifies symptoms of trauma because each encounter with race-related stress or trauma, whether it is personal or vicarious, leads to more stress. When this stress is magnified by the lack of opportunity to recover before the next experience, it intensifies. Ongoing exposure to racial microaggressions and vicarious experiences can be contributing factors to the development of chronic psychological distress and trauma and can lead to PTSD.

It is still unknown how prevalent PTSD is, but what can be said is that, in the United States, most ethnic and racial minority groups have higher rates of PTSD as compared with non-Hispanic Whites, and they may even experience PTSD symptoms of greater severity. Research has shown that discrimination plays a role in this disparity. For example, studies have shown that African American veterans show as much as 45 percent higher rates of PTSD as compared with White veterans (Carter 2007). One research study indicated that 37 percent of the Asian American veterans studied had PTSD, and that race-related stress was a stronger predictor of PTSD than exposure to combat (Loo *et al.* 2001). Carter theorizes that higher rates of diagnosed PTSD in non-White racial groups can be attributed to underlying, unacknowledged, and unaddressed race-based traumatic stress injuries (Carter *et al.* 2017).

It is not uncommon for people who have been exposed to ethnic and race-based stress and trauma over a lifetime, as well as historical trauma, to be unaware of its impact. Coping with the realities of living in a racially hostile and discriminatory environment teaches you to tune it out. Because the definition of PTSD has been limited to experiences of life-threatening events, people going through the daily lived experiences of racial wounding think they have to be able to identify one event in order for it to meet the criteria of a traumatic experience. To further complicate things, the clinical definition of PTSD, as well as its treatment, is embedded in European perspectives that tend to lack cultural relevance to people of other cultures, races, and ethnicities (Comas-Díaz *et al.* 2019).

It was not until I attended a workshop, only a few years ago, called Self-Care in the Face of Secondary Trauma, sponsored by the Association of Black Psychologists, that I realized my elementary school and college experiences were more than emotionally painful and stressful. They were actually traumatic. Recognizing that helped me better understand why it had taken me so long to recover from the emotional wounds I suffered. In one of the first workshops I conducted on Restorative Yoga for race-based stress and trauma, one of the participants said it took her about one month after the immersion to realize that it was the cumulative impact of many experiences of race-related events, experienced over a lifetime, which she had repressed, that was responsible for much of her previously unacknowledged emotional pain and suffering.

HIGH-EFFORT COPING

In her book *Becoming* (Obama 2018), Michelle Obama, the former First Lady of the United States, describes "marching to the beat" of unending effort to achieve an outcome, and a willingness to endure misery to look good in the eyes of others. A self-described high achiever, this is a coping style she relied on, beginning in childhood, to prove her worth, overcome obstacles to success, and to gain access to opportunities. The behavior she describes actually has a name. It is called high-effort coping and is not unique. It is a behavioral style that those who are locked out of opportunities, due to racial and ethnic discrimination, tend to utilize to gain access and to prove their worth. Researcher and epidemiologist Sherman James suggested that high-effort coping is a behavioral phenomenon, going all the way back to the Civil War, that African Americans engaged in after Emancipation, to overcome psychosocial barriers to equality (James 1994). According to James, high-effort coping was an attempt on the part of newly freed men and women to form an American identity by adopting and incorporating the dominant cultural beliefs, values, and behaviors of freedom, hard work, and self-reliance. In addition, it was an attempt to peacefully resist the new forms of oppression that recently 'freed' people were being subjected to. He coined the term "John Henryism" to describe the phenomenon because it reminded him of the legend of John Henry, an American folk hero.

According to the legend, John Henry was born into slavery, and after Emancipation became a laborer driving steel for the C&O Railroad. Steel drivers were those workers who hammered steel into rock to make holes for explosives that blasted the rock so that a railroad tunnel could be constructed. As the story goes, John Henry was a giant of a man with superhuman strength, considered to be the strongest, fastest, and hardest worker on the rails. The legend tells us that in a man-against-machine contest to drill a hole through a mountain, to make way for a tunnel, John Henry, with only a nine-pound hammer in his hands, beat the mechanical drill. But when he hammered his way through the mountain and got to the other side, he collapsed from exhaustion. His heart gave out and he died with his hammer in his hands (Nelson 2006).

In his research on health disparities between African Americans and European Americans, James found that due to the physical exertion of hard work and the prolonged effort to overcome and eliminate psychosocial barriers to success and equality, the African American population is disproportionately vulnerable to stress-related illness, including cardiovascular disease, hypertension, metabolic disease, and depression. He posits that the combined pressures of the psychological stresses associated with living in a racialized culture, feeling unsafe, and living on the edge of constant fear, along with doing the hard work of trying to overcome barriers to success, make one's body more susceptible to disease (James 1994).

Leith Mullings coined the term "Sojourner Syndrome" to explain a similar, but gender-specific, high-effort coping behavioral strategy that Black women employ. She called it the Sojourner Syndrome because the behavior is similar to the extraordinary efforts made by Sojourner Truth to resist and overcome racial and gender oppression. Sojourner Truth was born into slavery around 1799. After she became a free woman in 1827, she transformed herself from a domestic servant into an abolitionist itinerant preacher. She began traveling across the country to share her message of empowerment, exemplifying both resilience and resistance against oppression and adversity. In 1851 she gave a speech, commonly referred to as "Ain't I a Woman," at a women's convention held in Akron, Ohio. Her speech addressed the responsibilities of African American women that required them to work like men, to constantly ignore the stress of racial and gender discrimination, and to serve others at the expense of their own health (Painter 1996).

Mullings's research helped demonstrate that because of this active coping style, Black women, regardless of educational and socioeconomic status, are at higher risk of reproductive health consequences as compared with White women (Mullings 2005). Sojourner Syndrome is characterized by an obligation to be strong no matter what; to suppress displays of emotion; to be stoic in the face of physical and emotional pain; to be fiercely independent, not needing anyone and not asking for help; to succeed no matter what the obstacles or cost to her own health and well-being; and to put others' needs before her own (Mullings 2000). It is comparable to John Henryism in its determination to succeed through hard work and effort in spite of any barriers and obstacles, racial or otherwise, to equality and success. While this active coping style has survival value and can lead to financial, educational, and social gains, it comes at a high price for health and well-being.

It has already been established that racial discrimination is a chronic stressor that negatively affects the health of both men and women, including heart disease, cancer and stroke, and higher levels of mortality. But a particularly alarming report revealed that, according to the Centers for Disease Control and Prevention (CDC), heart disease and strokes cause one-third of pregnancy-related deaths, and that African American, Native American, and Alaska Native women are three times more likely to die of pregnancy-related causes than White women (Rabin 2019). Research has yet to determine if high-effort coping styles are linked to the risk factors associated with pregnancy-related mortality, but it is an area worthy of exploration.

I cannot speak with authority about other cultural norms, but I can speak with authority about African American cultural norms. John Henryism and the Sojourner Syndrome are culturally embedded values, part of ancestral memory. Most of us have heard some version of "In order to get half as far you have to do twice as much." High-effort coping is part of our DNA, so to speak, and is a cultural imperative that many, if not most, African Americans embody. On the positive side it can translate into excellence and resilience, but although engaging in this active coping style may give you a sense of control, a strong determination to succeed and excel, and a reluctance to ask for help, if you don't balance all that effort with ease, you are at risk for stress-related illnesses.

WHAT'S YOGA GOT TO DO WITH IT?

The Yoga Sutra is a collection of 196 aphorisms that describes the theory and practice of yoga, offering guidelines for spiritual growth and development, and how to live a meaningful, well-lived life. Sutra 2.16 (Desikachar 1995) tells us that the purpose of yoga is to alleviate pain and suffering, and to minimize it in the future. We know that all pain and suffering cannot be avoided, but we also know that certain yoga practices can relieve stress and can enhance the ability to process trauma. But one-size yoga does not fit all. Although there is research to indicate the efficacy of yoga to support PTSD (Van der Kolk 2014), to date there has been no research that identifies what form of yoga would be best suited to ease the distress of ethnic and race-based stress and trauma. However, Sutra 2.46 (Desikachar 1995) offers us some insight into a practice that might be effective. Yoga invites us to combine firmness with softness, stability with letting go, and rigor with ease. It teaches us not to strain, and at the same time asks us to develop the discipline of present-moment awareness and focused attention. Yoga offers a balance between ease and effort.

My hypothesis is that people who suffer from the ongoing stress and trauma of systemic oppression and daily experiences of racial wounding, and who engage in high-effort coping, can benefit from a practice that balances the nervous system by emphasizing ease. Restorative Yoga is presented as a practical self-care method for addressing the emotional wounds that result.

HOW RESTORATIVE YOGA CAN HELP

My first encounter with Ray was one year after his wife of five years had ended her life. He was still traumatized by her death and by the fact that she had taken her own life. He wanted some support as he went through the grieving process and the process of working through the trauma of her suicide. He was a high-achieving, successful businessman and a national leader in his field, honored for helping thousands of people rebuild their lives. He fit the profile of a person engaged in high-effort coping: a life dedicated to overcoming racial barriers to success, and to helping others recover from addiction. He worked non-stop to support others, sometimes neglecting his own needs. As I got to know him, it was evident that he was well defended against any feelings of vulnerability, making it nearly impossible for him to lower his defenses enough to complete the grieving process. In the beginning stages of his grieving and recovery from trauma, I introduced Restorative Yoga and meditation along with talk therapy, as part of our clinical treatment plan. After about six months, Ray announced that the Restorative Yoga and meditation were doing him more good than talk therapy and asked if we could just do that. He began attending the weekly group Restorative Yoga therapy classes I offered, and to this day swears by Restorative Yoga and meditation as self-care strategies that changed his life. He continues with his own practice and has now incorporated both Restorative Yoga and meditation into his work with people in recovery from alcohol and drug addiction.

Restorative Yoga is a receptive form of yoga that requires no physical exertion. To avoid stimulating the nervous system and to minimize stress and tension, it is practiced in stillness. Props such as blankets, bolsters, blocks, neck pillows, and eye masks are used to support the body as it remains in various yoga postures for extended periods of time. Breath is used to focus awareness and attention throughout the practice. The entire practice, from the very first pose to the very last one, is designed to stimulate the parasympathetic nervous system, the part of the involuntary nervous system that supports rest and recovery. In this practice you are actually working with the nervous system from the very first to the very last pose to evoke the relaxation response. You are not working with the traumatic event. You are working with the nervous system.

The relaxation response, a term coined by Herbert Benson, is the opposite of the stress response. It is a biologically innate response built into every human mind and body that can be accessed by focusing your awareness on your breath, or by silently repeating a word or a sound (mantra), and by repeatedly returning your awareness to your breath when you become distracted. Benson's research demonstrated that the relaxation response is characterized by a slower heart rate, slower metabolic rate, slower rate of breathing, lower blood pressure, and slower brain wave patterns, all of which support positive health outcomes (Benson 2000).

Many times when we sit down or lie down to relax, we fall asleep. But sleep is not always restful. When you are dealing with chronic stress and anxiety, your nervous system remains active, causing muscular tension even as you sleep. Because of this your body never fully relaxes. Restorative Yoga allows you to come into a state of deep rest without falling asleep, enabling you to notice where the body holds stress and tension and where it is relaxed. This is important because people who are chronically stressed are not always able to identify the difference between tension and relaxation, and don't realize that they can evoke the relaxation response on their own when they are tense or stressed. Observing and experiencing your body and mind shedding layers of stress and tension, which you may not have even known were there, is empowering.

The overall calming effect on the nervous system during a Restorative

Yoga practice creates conditions for the body's innate ability to restore itself. It rejuvenates, supports resilience by giving you an opportunity to recover before your next experience of stress, and prepares you for wise action. This is vitally important for people experiencing ongoing, cumulative, and recurrent stress or trauma. Because it is practiced in stillness, Restorative Yoga teaches you how to immobilize without fear. It supports feeling safe in stillness and increases alert awareness without hyper-vigilance. Learning safety in stillness is important for people who are in a continual state of high alert, constantly navigating danger, and always looking for an escape route. As you learn to navigate being safe through stillness, you are less likely to act out when you are under stress. The two young men arrested in the coffee shop who remained still, rather than resisting or protesting, are examples. Rather than acting on impulse, pausing first enables you to see with more clarity and make more deliberate and life-enhancing choices, both on and off your yoga mat. Restorative Yoga is an accessible self-care tool. Any body can do it and every body benefits from it. It can be practiced at home alone or in community. There are advantages to both, but an added benefit to practicing yoga with others in a group setting is the sense of belonging it offers (Novotney 2009).

THE YOGA OF RELATIONSHIP

We are hardwired for connection and motivated to avoid situations that exclude. Social exclusion, whether institutional, systemic or personal, conscious or unconscious, intentional or unintentional, is harmful, negatively affecting physical health and psychological well-being. Research has shown, for example, that people who have experienced the humiliation of social exclusion, and who report experiences of emotional loss and rejection early in childhood, are vulnerable to depression and to experiences of physical pain that have no medical explanation, such as fibromyalgia (Eisenberger 2012). Evolutionary history suggests that connection to others is beneficial because it increases our chances of survival by providing protection, safety, and additional resources. These findings should inspire us to think more carefully about the consequences of systematized, ongoing, recurrent ethnic and racial social exclusion and its impact.

As yogis, we have amazing tools that we can use to address ethnic and racial wounding and help the world become a better place for everyone. Yoga means union; the connection of body, mind, heart, and soul; the connection of one human being to another. It invites us into relationship with ourselves and with each other, even to those who are different from us. As the yoga community becomes more racially and ethnically diverse, we have an opportunity—actually, an obligation—to create welcoming communities that are culturally aware, supportive, and emotionally safe, and that promote social engagement and enhance well-being for all. But we have to work on ourselves first. This is an inside-out as well as an outside-in job. We live in a culture that is reactive to or in denial about issues associated with race and ethnicity, including cultural context. We have reflexive responses that might express as forms of social exclusion, shutting down a conversation, or minimizing someone else's pain in an effort to avoid dealing with our own. It can be as simple as diverting eye contact, which we may not think of as harmful but can actually be devastating.

Let me give you an example. A former client gave a TED Talk about her journey from abject poverty as a homeless, pregnant teenager eating out of garbage cans, to an abundant life as a well-respected Ph.D. university professor. Hers is a compelling story. But what I remember most about the story she told is this. She said the most painful experience of her life, while she was homeless, was the refusal of people to look at her, to see her, and acknowledge her humanity. In effect rendering her invisible.

Let us not make that mistake with each other. As aware yogis, let us do our part to ease the pain of ethnic and racial distress by intentionally practicing the yoga of relationship. Let us be in connection, and conversation with one another, eye to eye, heart to heart, and soul to soul, while honoring one another's humanity, regardless of racial and ethnic identity. Let this become our new culture. This is how we begin to heal the wounds of racial distress, and this is what yoga has to do with it.

REFLECTION

Delight in Stillness

What do you associate with being still? The mantra "If you want to get half as far, you have to do twice as much" is one that, if taken to heart, conflates doing the most with doing your best, and might result in concluding that resting in stillness is a waste of time and a form of laziness. As children, many of us were criticized and made to feel ashamed of being lazy or being selfish. "Go to your room!"

"Sit still until I tell you to move!" "You need a time out!" For those of us who grew up hearing these words when we misbehaved, is it any wonder that as adults we have an aversion to being still, to being quiet, or to being alone? Now add to these associations the stresses and traumatic experiences that keep us on high alert for the possibility of danger. When your nervous system is geared to looking out for danger, ready to take action at any moment, how likely is it that you will feel safe enough to remain still?

When being still is associated with laziness, punishment, or danger, it is understandable that you would be resistant to and unable to delight in stillness. No one wants to be judged as being selfish, lazy, bad, or to feel unsafe, so we keep busy. A lot of the time in our busy-ness we're not really accomplishing much; we're just busy being busy to avoid the unpleasantness we associate with being still. These associations are not necessarily conscious. But when you come to a place of stillness, tuning in to your body, your emotions, and your mind, letting go completely as you enter into a state of profound relaxation, your unconscious thoughts, memories, and emotions might come to the surface, and initially that can be disturbing. The good thing about that is that it allows you to become aware of what you associate with being still. This awareness helps you understand your resistance to taking the time to be still, both on and off your yoga mat.

Restorative Yoga teaches you to recognize what relaxation feels like. It teaches you that just because you're doing nothing doesn't mean nothing is happening. Your body is recalibrating, repairing, and rejuvenating. When you take care of your body, it takes care of you. Relaxation is not a waste of time, and the benefits are worth it. Decreases in heart rate, blood pressure, muscle tension, and anxiety are just some of the benefits. Relaxation also increases your energy level, stimulates memory, improves your ability to focus, enhances sleep, strengthens your immune system, and gives you an overall sense of well-being. Make time out a reward, not a punishment.

Many of us need to learn to associate stillness with something positive that is life-enhancing. In order to delight in stillness, we need to have positive and pleasant associations with being still. If you have trouble being still and relaxing unless you're asleep or distracted by television, music, or some other passive activity, here are some suggestions for making stillness a pleasant experience.

- Engage your imagination by visualizing a game from childhood that requires stillness. Freeze Tag, Statues, or Red Light/Green Light are some examples. Remembering how much fun that was can help you associate stillness with something joyful.
- Imagine all the good things you have to look forward to, or recall all the good things that have happened to you during the day.
- Remember a pleasant time of being still, a day alone on the beach enjoying the warmth of the sun with no place to go and nothing else to do.
- Envision holding a baby close to your heart, feeling his/her warmth, and synchronizing your breath and heartbeat with the baby's.
- Come up with your own version of what makes stillness a delight, and soon dropping into relaxation will become a pleasure.

DISCUSSION

In your daily life do you or have you experienced any of the following? How have these experiences impacted you?

- You are treated with less courtesy or respect than others.
- You receive poorer service than other people at restaurants or stores.
- You are treated as if you are not qualified or smart enough.
- People act as if they are afraid of you.
- You are intimidated, threatened, or harassed by authorities or associates.

Do you think this treatment is because of your race or ethnicity? Is there someone you can ask for emotional support when you need it?

REFERENCES

Benson, H. (2000) *The Relaxation Response*. New York, NY: HarperCollins.

Carter, R.T. (2007) "Racism and psychological and emotional injury: Recognizing and assessing race-based traumatic stress." *The Counseling Psychologist 35*, 13–105.

Carter, R.T., Johnson, V.E., Muchow, C., Lyons, J., Forquer, E., and Galgay, C. (2016) "Development of classes of racism measures for frequency and stress reactions: Relationship to race-based traumatic symptoms." *Traumatology 22*, 1, 63–74.

Carter, R.T., Johnson, V.E., Roberson, K., Krikinis, K., Mazzula, S.L., and Sant-Barket, S. (2017) "Race-based traumatic stress, racial identity statuses, and psychological functioning: An exploratory investigation." *Professional Psychology: Research and Practice 48*, 1, 30–37.

Carter, R.T., Mazzula, S., Rodolfo, V., Vazquez, R., *et al.* (2013) "Initial development of the Race-Based Traumatic Stress Symptom Scale: Assessing the impact of racism." *Psychological Trauma: Theory, Research, Practice, and Policy 5*, 1, 1–9.

Comas-Díaz, L., Hall, G.N., Neville, H.A., and Kazak, A.E. (eds.) (2019) "Racial trauma: Theory, research, and healing" [Special issue]. *American Psychologist 74*, 1.

Desikachar, T.K.V. (1995) *The Heart of Yoga: Developing a Personal Practice*. Rochester, VT: Inner Traditions International.

Eisenberger, N.I. (2012) "The neural bases of social pain: Evidence for shared representations with physical pain." *Psychosomatic Medicine 74*, 2, 126–135.

James, S.A. (1994) "John Henryism and the health of African Americans." *Culture, Medicine, and Psychiatry 18*, 163–182.

Loo, C.M., Fairbank, J.A., Scurfield, R.M., Ruch, L.O., *et al.* (2001) "Measuring exposure to racism: Development and validation of a race-related stressor scale (RRSS) for Asian American Vietnam veterans." *Psychological Assessment 13*, 503–520.

Mullings, L. (2000) "African American women making themselves: Notes on the role of black feminist research." *Souls: A Critical Journal of Black Politics, Culture, and Society 2*, 18–29. Accessed on 11/14/2019 at www.columbia.edu/cu/ccbh/souls/vol2no4/vol2num4art2.pdf.

Mullings, L. (2005) "Resistance and resilience: The Sojourner Syndrome and the social context of reproduction in central Harlem." *Transforming Anthropology 13*, 79–91.

Nelson, S.R. (2006) *Steel Drivin' Man: John Henry, the Untold Story of an American Legend*. New York, NY: Oxford University Press.

Novotney, A. (2009) "Yoga as a practice tool." *Monitor on Psychology 40*, 10, 38–42.

Obama, M. (2018) *Becoming*. New York, NY: Crown Publishing Group.

Painter, N.I. (1996) *Sojourner Truth: A Life, a Symbol*. New York, NY: W.W. Norton & Company.

Rabin, R.C. (2019) "Huge racial disparities found in deaths linked to pregnancy." *The New York Times*, May 7. Accessed on 11/14/2019 at www.nytimes.com/2019/05/07/health/pregnancy-deaths-.html.

Van der Kolk, B. (2014) *The Body Keeps the Score*. New York, NY: Penguin Books.

Chapter 3

THE HEALING POWER OF RELATIONSHIP

W E ARE social beings with a built-in need to feel connected and safe in our relationships. Safe relationships involve more than being tolerant. An attitude of tolerance carries with it the energy of endurance and indifference. "I am willing to put up with you because it's the right thing to do, but I am not inspired to engage you or to connect with you because I'm really not that interested in you"—that's tolerance. Safe connected relationships also involve more than offering support. They require mutuality and reciprocity, give and take. They are characterized by interpersonal communication that is attuned to and honors someone else's experience of the world.

In order to grow as a community, as the world of yoga becomes more ethnically and racially diverse, we have to be prepared to engage in constructive conversations with each other about race, ethnicity, and culture. Engaging with one another effectively on these emotionally loaded topics depends on each of us being aware of our own internal reactions regarding issues as they come up. It requires making our relationships with each other more important than the issues. It involves making a commitment to remain in conversation and connection, and to repair the inevitable ruptures that will occur when there is a misunderstanding. Agreeing to disagree does nothing to enhance connection because it truncates opportunities for greater understanding, growth, and intimacy. Remaining in communication for the purpose of understanding perspectives other than one's own supports all three. The ability to engage in these conversations respectfully and non-defensively, with openness and curiosity, strengthens our connection to each other.

At a lecture on yoga, art, and culture, the speaker, in an attempt to be humorous, made references to Indian culture that the South Asians in the audience experienced as misinformed and disrespectful. During the question-and-answer period, they offered the speaker feedback to correct any misunderstanding that may have been communicated to those in the audience unfamiliar with the culture. The speaker, who was not Indian, appeared to be offended by the feedback, became agitated and defensive, abruptly ended the discussion, and walked off the stage. Reactive, reflexive, and defensive responses are indications of some sort of pain and suffering of your own that you may not be aware of. Whatever you protect, defend, and avoid is an indication of an unhealed wound that prevents you from remaining calm and engaged, and from listening to what someone is trying to communicate. Approaching issues of ethnicity, race, and cultural differences is highly emotionally charged because of the unacknowledged and unhealed wounds that we carry within ourselves. In a racially and ethnically diverse culture, becoming culturally and racially attuned is an important skill for each of us to hone. Yoga has everything to teach us about how to connect to ourselves and to each other. It starts with compassionate self-study.

Unacknowledged and unaddressed stress and trauma affect your mood and your ability to be in attuned connection with others. Because ongoing stress and trauma keep you on high alert, you are prone to anxiety, irritability, and inflexibility, making it difficult to focus your attention, to listen, to think clearly, and to make good decisions. You are more easily triggered by minor irritations, causing you to be combative and attack, or withdrawn and shut down. Your ability to communicate effectively and to form and sustain bonds with others is compromised because you don't feel safe. Unhealed emotional wounds make attuned relationships problematic.

There's a story I like to share about the cost of ignoring our emotional wounds. A dog is lying on the ground next to his owner whimpering. A passerby asks, "What's wrong with your dog?" The owner says, "He's lying on a nail." The passerby asks, "Well, why doesn't he get up?" The owner says, "Because that hurts even more." If you've ever stepped on a sharp object, you know that in order for healing to occur you have to extract it. Sometimes that hurts more than stepping on it did, and so it is understandable that you might resist pulling it out. But leaving it in is never helpful and does more harm than good. Even though removing the object may hurt more than stepping on it did, the pain of removal is temporary, whereas tolerating or ignoring pain retards the healing process and makes matters worse. This is true of both physical and emotional pain. In order to heal, the dog has to get up off the nail even though that hurts more than lying on it does. In order for us to heal, as it pertains to race and ethnicity, each of us needs to get up off the nail of our own combativeness, defensiveness, hyper-vigilance, and fragility. If we don't, healing cannot occur, and we risk becoming blind, numb, indifferent, and even cruel in the face of our own and others' pain and suffering.

Resilience in the face of ethnic and race-based stress and trauma is critical to physical and emotional health and well-being. Resilience is the capacity to recover quickly and bounce back from ongoing, cumulative, and recurrent stress before it becomes chronic or traumatic, or before you burn out. Individuals with strong emotional support are more resilient in the face of stress and social exclusion than those who experience the isolation of social exclusion without support. Rather than eliciting the fight-or-flight response, relational connection elicits the tend-and-befriend response. To tend and befriend is to reach out to others for comfort when you are in distress rather than to fight, avoid, or withdraw. Reaching out to others in times of distress has a calming effect and there is a biochemical reason for this. When we are in positive connection with others, oxytocin, a neurochemical associated with empathy, love, and relationship building, is active in the body, sending internal signals that reduce the fight–flight or the withdraw–shutdown response. Think for a moment about how you feel when someone smiles, makes eye contact, and greets you warmly. Think about times when someone just listens to you without offering advice or making suggestions. Think about the times when you smile, make eye contact, and greet someone else warmly. Think about the times when you are able to listen to someone without offering advice or making suggestions. How do you feel? How do they respond?

SAFETY IN VULNERABILITY

Racial and ethnic wounds are highly charged and deeply emotional. Because of that we have to feel safe enough within ourselves and in relationship to other people to engage and remain in constructive discussions about race and ethnicity. We have to be willing to be vulnerable and to feel safe in our vulnerability. Creating safety in vulnerability starts with creating a safe and welcoming internal holding environment. What that means is practicing self-acceptance and engaging in compassionate self-study, honoring the best in us with humility, and admitting our flaws without shame, blame, or criticism. We learn safety in vulnerability first by cultivating a discipline of loving kindness toward ourselves. This allows us to view ourselves with compassion for our errors, and to forgive ourselves for our mistakes. When we can do this for ourselves, we can do it for others. We are pretty clear about creating externally safe holding environments, but how much time do we take to create safe internal holding environments? We tend to be a self-critical culture. We're used to shame, blame, and criticism as our companions. Self-compassion practices are relevant to easing our suffering and enable us to become self-reflective without beating up on ourselves.

A safe internal holding space has to be constructed; it doesn't just happen. We build it from the ground up. The foundation is built by finding a way into your personal inner sanctum in a way that arouses tenderness, warmth, and friendliness toward yourself. Yoga practices can teach us how to do that. For example, you can begin by entering into meditation with a sense of wonder and curiosity in a warm, friendly, welcoming way.

- Begin your meditation by simply asking yourself, "I wonder what will come up for me today?"
- Next, greet yourself by asking, "How are you today?" Wait for an answer.
- Follow this with, "What do you need right now?" Wait for an answer.
- Place both hands over your heart center and settle in.
- Silently repeat to yourself: "May I be safe. May I be at ease. May I be at peace."
- A self-compassion meditation can follow.

Creating a safe internal holding environment for your meditation supports you in observing your mind with interest from a place of awareness, clear perception, and loving kindness. When you are able to observe the mind from this vantage point, you are more inclined to stick with the practice and are better able to tolerate the fluctuations of mind you will encounter. You begin to notice that the mind is always in flux, and that the thoughts that arise are random and not necessarily trustworthy. Because you have created a safe internal holding space, instead of being self-critical as you observe your mind, it begins to dawn on you that just because you think something does not mean you have to believe it or act on what it's telling you. Should you trust a mind that is unexamined? Should you trust a mind that is always changing? Should you act on what it tells you, or is it better to wait until you experience a sense of calm that supports clarity and wisdom before you act?

Sutra 1.2 (Desikachar 1995) tells us that yoga is the practice of focusing your awareness without being distracted by your fluctuating thoughts, in order to cultivate clarity of mind. Clarity of mind keeps you from acting on thoughts that can be full of misapprehension. Yoga teaches you that you do not have to believe your thoughts; it teaches you to occupy the seat of awareness, to observe your mind, to be fully present, and to exercise discernment before you take action. It teaches you to pause and look within to cultivate clear perception first. Dealing with issues of race and ethnicity can trigger all kinds of thoughts and knee-jerk reactions. Compassionate self-study supported by a loving-kindness meditation practice is invaluable.

FEAR OF OTHERS

On a lovely summer evening, my husband, son, and I were returning home from a family dinner. We were happy, laughing, and enjoying one another's company. Since we live in different parts of the country, we had not been together for a while, so for us it was a special occasion. As we approached our condominium, a neighbor, whom we had never met, was opening the gate to the complex to leave just as we were putting our key in the lock to come in. He looked startled when he saw us, as if we did not belong there. Without smiling, he said, "I'll assume you're not criminals and let you in." Now this may have been a perfectly innocent remark, but I suspect it was a culturally conditioned one, one that associates black and brown skin tones with criminality. It may seem like an innocuous remark if you have never been stereotyped, but it triggered all of us because African Americans, particularly males, are commonly and dangerously stereotyped as criminals. My husband kept his composure and responded by saying, "You're right, we're not criminals. We are a physician, a psychologist, and an attorney." Looking sheepish, without saying anything else, the man moved on. Did our neighbor understand why he greeted us the way he did? Did he have any idea of the emotional impact his remarks had? Why didn't he just smile and say, "Good evening?" Was he too afraid? Of what? Why was he unable to maintain eye contact? Did he ask himself any of these questions?

We feel frightened when we feel endangered. When it comes to race and ethnicity, there are those who are afraid and those who are feared. Which group do you identify with? Depending on the context, most likely both. When it comes to examining your thoughts about race and ethnicity, it is important to be honest with yourself. Are you or have you ever been afraid of cultures, races, or ethnicities different from your own? Are you or have you ever been afraid to be near people who are not similar to you? Do you jump to conclusions or carry stereotypes about people whom you see as different? Do you avoid going to places where people who are not like you congregate in large groups? If so, why? The next question is: Where does your fear of others come from? Is it coming from your internalized expectations and biases, or is there really a threat to your safety? Are you reacting from present-moment awareness, some remembered trauma from your past, or a culturally biased understanding of who is a threat and who is not? Are you reacting to an external threat or an internal trigger? As part of self-study, these are important questions to ask yourself.

FIRST LOOK WITHIN

In 2016 I was a guest on an internationally syndicated medical lifestyle show. The topic was race, ethnicity, and hate crimes. It was at a time when police killings of unarmed Black men and women and hate crimes toward ethnic and religious minorities were on the rise in the United States. Global animus was growing toward refugees seeking asylum from poverty, violence, and war in their own countries, and racial and ethnic enmity were on the rise worldwide. I was asked to share my thoughts on what motivates people to commit hate crimes. I explained that all human beings, regardless of race and ethnicity, need and want to love, be loved, and to feel safe. When those needs are frustrated, people become fearful. If they remain fearful long enough, they become angry. Prolonged periods of anger can morph into hatred, and once that happens, you lose touch with the human need for love, kindness, and compassion and begin to act out of hatred. People who act out of hatred tend to demonize difference, making it evil, awful, and wrong, and that just reinforces fear. The host asked, "How do we break out of that?" I explained that the first step is to recognize how far down the path toward hatred you have traveled and then trace the path backward until you get back to your basic need to love, be loved, and feel safe. If you get all the way to hatred, start there and go backward. Ask yourself, "What am I angry about?" Answer it. Then ask yourself, "What am I afraid of?" Answer it. Then ask yourself, "What do I really need?" The assumption is that you will eventually realize the primal human need, to love, be loved, and to feel safe. The hope is that you begin acting in ways that will reflect that, and that you will be able to extend that to people regardless of race or ethnicity. Hatred and love are not just feelings. Both are choices. Realizing that is the first step toward change. You can choose to stay on the pathway toward hatred or you can choose the pathway toward love. I have just described the way back to love.

The process I describe requires a degree of self-awareness, self-reflection, and self-regulation. When we feel threatened, it is a split-second reaction and is frequently met with a split-second response. Taking your time is not what most people are inclined to do when they are afraid. What I suggested takes time, requires practice and maybe even professional guidance and support. While we each have the capacity for self-reflection, not everyone is practiced in using it. If you are self-reflective when you become frightened, you will ask yourself, "What about this is scaring me?" A person who is acting out of fear and who is not self-reflective will likely conclude, "You've scared me. You're the problem, and I'm going to defend myself against you." Once that conclusion is reached, interpersonal connection is ruptured and whatever action you take is unlikely to be wise, constructive, or helpful. The problem is, when you act out of fear or anger, the feelings do not go away and you continue to project these emotions onto the next person or situation. This is why it is important to understand that just because you're feeling threatened, it does not mean you are being threatened. You may be reacting to internal triggers, not to a real threat of danger. But how can you know for sure? Understanding the physiology of emotion can help.

THE PHYSIOLOGY OF EMOTION

The polyvagal theory, developed by Stephen Porges, explains our emotional reactions from a mind–body perspective (Porges 2011). The theory explains the role the nervous system plays in triggering our sense of danger and the role it plays in restoring a sense of safety. It explains the ever-present, ongoing threat detection feature of the nervous system that operates on an instinctive level. It explains how one nervous system affects another through co-regulation. Additionally, it explains the importance of cultivating a resilient nervous system so that instead of acting out when you are triggered by fear or anger, you can engage with others in ways that support feelings of safety. Viewing ethnic and race-based stress and trauma through the lens of the polyvagal theory sheds light on the role attuned relationships can play in supporting a healthy, balanced nervous system that can mediate reactivity associated with ethnic and race-related events.

The nervous system is composed of two parts: one part is within your conscious control, like waving your hand or lifting your arm, and one part operates outside of conscious awareness. The part that you cannot control is called the autonomic nervous system (ANS). The ANS has two branches: the sympathetic branch that is associated with our fight-or-flight response, and the parasympathetic branch that is associated with our rest-and-digest, tend-and-befriend response. The two systems alternate to support health and well-being, and are associated with regulating our immune system, our ability to sleep and relax, and our digestion. The function of the autonomic nervous system is to help you survive when you are in danger, and to help you flourish and grow when you feel safe. The ANS is connected to every organ in your body and affects all of the bodily functions that you do not control such as your heartbeat, body temperature, blood pressure, digestive system, metabolism, and breath. It acts as an internal safety monitor that is always scouting for cues of danger and safety. Its job is to keep you alive. Your autonomic state affects your sense of safety and your ability to connect with others.

The typical approach to explaining the autonomic nervous system is to describe the parasympathetic and sympathetic branches being in opposition to each other—that is, when one is turned on, the other is turned off. In other words, when the parasympathetic system is stimulated, you are relaxed, and when the sympathetic system is activated, you are stressed. Polyvagal theory offers a new understanding of how the nervous system works. There are actually three autonomic states associated with the nervous system: a state of safety, a state of defense, and a state of collapse. Each state is part of the evolutionary development of the nervous system and has its own unique response in service of keeping you safe and alive (Porges 2011). When your nervous system is regulated and resilient, you move back and forth between the states of the nervous system as necessary. When the sympathetic and parasympathetic branches are working together, you are in homeostasis and experience a sense of safety and well-being.

EVOLUTION OF THE NERVOUS SYSTEM

The most ancient part of the nervous system is one that we share with our reptilian ancestors who, when under threat, immobilized and played dead to remain undetected and safe. Like reptiles, in the case of extreme danger or life threat, we freeze and shut down to survive. This is what happens in trauma. The next evolutionary development in the nervous system involved movement to defend against threat. When we get triggered by a sense of danger, adrenaline and cortisol are released into the body to help us take action. The rush of adrenaline makes it hard to be still, think clearly, and make good choices, so the actions we take in this state of autonomic arousal are not always wise or effective, and can do more harm than good. The most recent evolutionary development in the mammalian nervous system is called the social engagement system. It involves a sense of calm and well-being that comes from being in attuned connection with others. The nervous system evolved to support feelings of safety and to ensure survival through attuned, supportive, and loving relationships. When feeling threatened, in order to restore a sense of safety, the nervous system works in a hierarchical fashion. It recruits the most recently evolved social engagement feature first. If that does not work, the fight–flight feature activates, and, in extreme situations, the most primitive feature, the freeze response clicks in (Porges 2011).

Each autonomic state—safety, defense, and collapse—follows a certain pathway. The sympathetic branch, located in the middle of the spinal cord, is the pathway that detects signs of threat, and releases adrenaline and cortisol into your system to prepare you for taking action to protect yourself. It is the fight–flight response. The parasympathetic branch of the nervous system (PNS) can be recruited to calm us when we are aroused, or to shut us down when we fear for our lives. It involves two pathways that travel through the vagus nerve.

The vagus nerve is the longest nerve in the body and plays a role in regulating heart rate, blood pressure, digestion, perspiration, auditory signals, vocalization, and facial expression. It travels downward from the brain stem, linking the lungs, heart, diaphragm, and stomach to the brain, and travels back up to the brain, connecting to the nerves in the neck, throat, eyes, and ears. Because it travels in two directions, the vagus nerve allows the brain and body to transmit information back and forth, from top to bottom and bottom to top, communicating about various bodily functions. In mammals there are two vagal circuits: the ancient unmyelinated circuit, called the dorsal vagal circuit, that detects extreme danger and cues of life threat, and the newer myelinated circuit called the ventral vagal circuit, also called the social engagement system, that picks up on cues of safety. The two circuits attach at separate locations in the brain stem.

The dorsal vagal pathway connects to the organs below the diaphragm including the stomach, spleen, liver, kidneys, and large intestines. It is the pathway that in the case of extreme danger or life threat causes us to protect ourselves by disengaging and shutting down. When this happens, there are actual physiological shifts that impair the ability to hear conversation and instead attune to hearing sounds of danger. Eyelids droop, eye contact is avoided, the facial muscles go slack, flattening out facial expression, and the pain threshold increases, sometimes causing feelings of numbness. When this part of the nervous system is activated, we may faint, or dissociate, all in service of protecting ourselves and keeping us alive. Like our reptilian ancestors, our nervous system tries to protect us by playing dead. This response is extreme, the response of last resort, and is associated with trauma.

The ventral vagal pathway connects above the diaphragm to the heart, lungs, throat, inner ear, and the facial muscles around the mouth and eyes. It is the pathway to feeling safe and socially engaged. In this state you are able to smile, make eye contact, speak in soothing tones, and listen to conversation. You feel creative and playful in this state, can laugh at yourself and with others, and you can enjoy your own company without suffering from loneliness. You have an overall sense of well-being that you actually feel physically. The ventral vagal pathway has an inhibitory influence, which Porges calls the vagal brake, that regulates heartbeat and keeps it from racing (Porges 2011). When the parasympathetic nervous system detects cues of safety, the vagal brake is on, oxytocin is released into the body, and we are able to rest, relax, and experience compassion, empathy, and deep connection within ourselves and with others. The vagal brake also keeps the sympathetic fight–flight part of the nervous system in check. When the nervous system detects cues that cause you to feel threatened, either because you are in danger of harm or because you perceive that you are, the vagal brake releases, your heart rate increases, and your sympathetic system dominates.

Since the nervous system evolved to work from the top down, the social engagement system is recruited as our first line of defense. Instead of reacting to whatever threat we are experiencing by running from it or fighting, we attempt to restore safety through connection. We smile, make eye contact, and speak in well-modulated, soothing tones. When this line of defense does not work or would not be wise, the vagal brake releases, the sympathetic fight–flight response takes over, and we take action to protect and defend ourselves to re-establish safety. It is only in cases of extreme danger that the most ancient and primitive nervous system defense is recruited, and we move into a physiological state of collapse, just as our reptilian ancestors did when they played dead to protect themselves.

When the nervous system picks up cues of safety, we are able to engage with others in a friendly, non-threatening way. When it picks up cues of danger, the nervous system automatically prepares the body to take whatever action is necessary to be safe and survive. It moves, it fights, it protects. This is a dynamic system that changes as needed. We are not intended to remain in just one state or the other. We navigate between states of social engagement and mobilization. When the nervous system is operating in an efficient manner, we are able to bounce back from a defensive state to a state of safety in a short period of time. The ability to alternate between social engagement and mobilization as needed is a measure of resilience. We need a resilient nervous system and a toned vagus for that to occur.

ACTING OUT

The nervous system evaluates risk by detecting non-verbal cues of what is going on around you. It tunes in to sounds, body language, facial expressions, and how close or far away someone is in relationship to you. Think about the times when someone gets too close to you physically. You feel uncomfortable and feel an impulse to move, to get away, or to strike out. It is an involuntary impulse. While you have no choice about the nervous system's instinctive response, with awareness you do have a choice about what to do when it clicks in. A defensive reaction can be triggered by something as simple as someone placing their yoga mat too close to yours. This is not rational but is an instinctive response. You feel it in your body. Remember, this is not a cognitive process; it is a felt experience. My reaction when a yoga teacher first massaged my neck and touched my head in savasana is an example. The first thing I felt was tension and an impulse to get away. At the same time, I could sense by the teacher's touch that it was a loving not a hostile touch, and I was able to remain still even though I felt uncomfortable. Over time, by remaining still and resisting the impulse to react, I was able to receive being touched with present-moment awareness, and was able to realize that no one was trying to hurt or humiliate me. It took some time, but eventually my internal experience changed.

Neuroception is the term coined by Porges to describe this instinctive response. It is not a choice, nor is it within our conscious control. It operates without any thought and causes shifts in the autonomic nervous system, moving you into a state of defense without any awareness of what triggers it (Buczynski and Porges 2015). The nervous system has its own intelligence and assesses the situation and then initiates a response. After that happens, and it happens instantly, the meaning-making part of us clicks in and we make up a story to match the response. You may have heard the expression "We see the world as we are, not as it actually is." What this means is that what you are seeing in the outside world almost always matches the stories you are telling yourself, based on the state of your nervous system.

But here's the thing: neuroception doesn't always get it right. In states of chronic stress—that is, stress that is outside of your awareness—or in trauma, the nervous system's ability to pick up on cues of safety or danger is compromised and you may not be able to tell the difference between actual danger and a trigger of danger. You might also think you are safe when you're not. Under the influence of stress or trauma you become biased toward seeing danger where there is none, or you can be blind to cues of actual danger and think you're safe when you're not. In the case of race and ethnicity, based on Western civilization's cultural conditioning, there is a bias toward seeing non-White people as dangerous and White people as safe. Because we are meaning-making beings, who need explanations and reasons for why we are reacting the way we are, we make up stories to match our nervous system's response. The story does not come first; it comes after the nervous system sends a signal.

When you don't feel safe, you make up a story that says that the person, or the situation you are in, is the threat. When you feel safe, you make up a story that matches your feeling of safety. What this means is that whatever story you're telling yourself supports the nervous system's response. It might result in taking aggressive action toward someone when it's unwarranted or giving the benefit of the doubt when it's unwarranted. Repeating the story over and over again, being bombarded with images or surrounded by people that reinforce your story trains your nervous system to respond accordingly. Think about the manager of the coffee shop, and the college student who called the police to report someone, not because they were in any danger, but because of the internal triggers they were responding to. Think about the referee who acted aggressively toward the high school student by insisting that his dreadlocks be cut off, even though the student tried to cooperate by agreeing to wear headgear to cover his hair. Think about the messages you have been exposed to through stories and images that tell you who is dangerous and who is safe, based on cultural norms. All of this informs your nervous system's responses.

SELF-REGULATION

The coffee-shop manager and the college student who called the police appeared to feel threatened even though no one was threatening them. The actions of the referee were clearly hostile, even though the student tried to cooperate by agreeing to wear headgear to cover his hair. Where was their fear and hostility coming from? Were they responding to an internal trigger or an external threat? Calling the police to report someone who is not actually threatening you suggests the inability to detect the difference between an internal trigger and an external threat. It also demonstrates an inability to manage your own fear and agitation. Forcing someone to change their appearance or insisting that someone be removed from your presence, just because you don't like the way they look, suggests the inability to recognize your internal triggers and an inability to manage your own hostility. Relying on an external solution, such as calling the police or forcing someone to have his hair cut off, to solve an internal problem never works and is harmful and dangerous.

When our nervous system fails us, we act out (Buczynski and Porges 2015). When it serves us, we are able to navigate out of a perceived threat without acting out. As a necessary survival skill, when you are faced with threat on an ongoing basis, you learn to navigate out rather than acting out in the face of danger. When you know that you are perceived as a threat, for example, you are not as easily triggered because you've learned how to navigate out of danger and into safety, not for anyone else's benefit but for your own. When you aren't practiced emotionally in maneuvering out of threatening situations, you are more prone to acting out.

Witnesses to the coffee-shop arrest said they would have exploded in anger if they had been treated the way the two young men who were arrested were treated. Michelle Saahene, the young woman who first brought attention to the fact that the young men were being racially profiled, pointed out to the onlookers that that is because protesting in anger did not pose a threat to their safety. Contrast that with the response of the two young men arrested who said in an interview that, despite fearing for their lives, they were able to hold themselves in check and remain alert and present to the real danger they were in, and act accordingly. They did not resist or protest their treatment because they knew that doing so was perilous. The high school wrestler who was forced to have his hair cut off before his wrestling match was reportedly visibly shaken, but in spite of that fought and won his match. These are examples of the ability to successfully self-regulate in the face of hostility and potential life threat. But here's the problem. When you become an expert in navigating out of danger, you are also at risk of burning out. You need opportunities to recalibrate. Self-reflective awareness, attuned relationships, and yoga practices that support ease can help to do that.

To summarize, the nervous system can be activated by external events that are actual threats to physical or emotional safety, or by internal conditioning that is based on cultural norms, beliefs, past experience, ancestral memory, and the stories you tell yourself. In other words, the fear response can be turned on by an external threat or by an internal trigger. What is important to understand is this. The nervous system does not know the difference between an internal trigger and an external threat, and goes into a fight, flight, or shutdown response automatically. In a state of hyper-arousal (fight–flight) we find ourselves using strategies of confrontation or avoidance in an attempt to re-establish a sense of safety. In a state of hypo-arousal (freeze–immobilization) we use strategies of withdrawal, dissociation, and shutdown in an attempt to re-establish safety. These are adaptive responses to stress and trauma. When we remain stuck in these states of hyper-arousal or hypo-arousal, we are in states of dysregulation, unable to discern with clarity when we are safe and when we are not, as well as unable to access our social engagement system, our safe connection to others, to re-establish a sense of safety.

You are not in control of your instinctive response. What is within your control is learning to know the difference between an internal trigger and an external threat and learning to behave accordingly. Your level of awareness, the way you think, and how resilient your nervous system is all influence how you respond when you feel threatened. You are in charge of that. Cultivating attuned relationships, engaging in meditative practices, and practicing Restorative Yoga are examples of what you can do to tone your nervous system, keep it healthy, and support resilience.

EYE TO EYE, HEART TO HEART, KNEE TO KNEE...

Whenever I begin a workshop, no matter how large or how small the group is, we sit in a circle and I invite people to introduce themselves to the entire group by name and to share what brings them to the workshop and what they hope to learn. If the group is too large for that to be practical, in the interest of time, I break them up into small groups and have them do it there. This is a way to invite people to begin relating to one another. It serves as a warm-up for going into a deeper level of connection where we sit in pairs, cross-legged on the floor (unless a chair would be more comfortable), facing each other eye to eye, heart to heart, and knee to knee. We sit facing each other in silence for about one minute. This is a non-verbal way to establish connection and to initiate feeling safe in relationship to one another. At first it seems awkward and maybe even uncomfortable, because we're not speaking to each other, and because we're not used to engaging in this way, but gradually an internal shift occurs and people settle in. The shift is actually an internal shift in our physiology. When one settled body encounters another, a deeper settling of both nervous systems occurs. We are beginning to establish a mutually safe relational holding environment. The next step in this exercise is to support reciprocity by engaging in the following exchange. Whoever goes first says to their partner, "I am breathing in just like you." The partner responds by saying, "You are breathing in just like me." Next, the first person says, "I am breathing out just like you." The partner responds, "You are breathing out just like me." In the final exchange the first person says, "We are breathing in and out together." The partner responds, "We are breathing in and out together." Then they switch and the second person begins the same exchange. After both partners exchange, we pause and once more sit in silence across from one another before we share with each other what we experienced in the exercise. Usually, there is a marked difference in the experience at the end of the exchange than at the beginning. This is because we have embodied reciprocity and mutuality through the exercise, and our nervous systems have begun to co-regulate. What that means is that your autonomic state has synchronized with another autonomic state, creating a felt sense of safety between the two of you.

When one viscerally calm nervous system encounters another, a deeper sense of calm can occur in both nervous systems. By the same token, when one agitated nervous system encounters another, the agitation can lodge in both nervous systems and the opportunity for connection is diminished. In order to feel safe, we need opportunities for connection with each other. In order for this to happen, we need to feel safe with each other; without this we suffer (Buczynski and Porges 2012). We live in a global community of difference, and whether you are aware of it or not, what affects one of us affects all of us. This means that even though we may be living geographically and socially segregated lives, we each have a responsibility to regulate our own autonomic state so that we can reach out and offer cues of safety to each other regardless of racial, ethnic, or cultural differences. We have to be willing to show up safe for one another. Reciprocity in relationship is enlivening and creates a sense of safety. Our sense of safety comes from within, not from the removal of threat, which only builds barriers and reinforces fear. Being in connection reinforces a feeling of safety. By introducing elements of play, warmth, friendliness, curiosity, wonder, and caring attention, a yoga class can be a relational holding environment where healing body, mind, and spirit can occur. This was the experience I had in a Restorative Yoga class I took to manage a physical injury with a teacher who is a master of relational connection.

THE POWER OF PRESENCE

Years ago I slipped and fell on a patch of ice and landed flat on my back on a concrete sidewalk. It really hurt. Fortunately, I did not require medical intervention. At the time I was practicing an active form of yoga asana and was not able to continue because of the back injury. A few days after the accident, one of my yoga teachers called and said, "I heard you hurt your back in a fall. I think I can help you with that." I'm pretty certain the healing process began with that phone call. The kindness and compassion in his voice, and just the act of his reaching out to me, caused me to feel a deep sense of relief and gratitude. I could literally feel myself relax and let go of some of the tension caused by the fall. I attended his Restorative Yoga class and he put me in a supported Supta Baddha Konasana right away. If you are unfamiliar with the posture, you can find a description and an image of it in Chapter 8. Normally, this is a pose that you might hold no longer than 20 minutes. It releases tension in and around the hips, opens your chest and diaphragm to support deep diaphragmatic breathing, and promotes emotional and physical relaxation and restoration.

The teacher and I laugh about it now, but he let me stay in the pose for the entire hour, not because he planned to but because it was apparent to him that the pose was doing its job. I went into a deep state of rest and relaxation, different from sleep, where healing could occur. While the pose was indeed restful and relaxing, there was something else going on. The state of deep rest I experienced was aided by virtue of the teacher's ability to non-verbally communicate a deep and genuine sense of caring and concern by his presence alone. Never underestimate the power of presence. The most powerful teachers and therapists are those who can model authentic presence and bring it to their work, inviting and allowing another person to have his or her experience just as it is. What a person's wounded places need most is for someone to be there with them. They don't need anyone to diagnose, heal, or fix the problem, to tell them how sorry they are that they got hurt or that everything is going to be all right. They need the full presence of your being, which is itself the healing balm. This is true whether a person's pain is physical or emotional.

Being present for someone in the face of their pain and suffering can be challenging. This is certainly true in the face of ethnic and race-based stress and trauma. Regardless of race and ethnicity, most of us get triggered by our own unconscious, unexamined, and unhealed racial wounds. When that happens, the sympathetic nervous system responds and we feel an impulse to say or do something. This is where the wisdom "Don't just do something, sit there" applies. There is a time for doing something and a time for doing nothing. Presence is the recognition of the power of doing nothing and instead just being. Practicing stillness through meditative practices and Restorative Yoga helps us hone the skill. Learning to be present keeps us out of reactivity. The impulse to be helpful and do something to alleviate someone else's pain often comes from the need to protect ourselves from feeling our own suffering. Your emotional reactivity is never helpful. This is why help is not always helpful.

The therapeutic techniques we use are important but secondary. That was certainly the case in my situation. What came first was the teacher's ability to be present with me in my suffering. His presence helped me feel safe and well taken care of enough to let go and relax into a healing process. Can you be present with someone in the face of race-based traumatic stress injury?

REMEMBERED WELLNESS

The body has an intelligence of its own independent of the thinking mind and knows how to heal itself. Dr. Herbert Benson calls the ability to invoke feeling calm and non-reactive during stressful situations "remembered wellness" (Benson 1996). It is the most natural thing in the world. You cannot make it happen, and you don't have to, but you can create conditions that optimize the ability of the body to remember its innate blueprint of order, balance, harmony, and flow.

Restorative Yoga stimulates the parasympathetic nervous system, strengthens vagal tone, and makes it easier for the body to relax after stress. It buffers the nervous system and supports you in feeling safe in stillness. Feeling safe in stillness is an experience that people who are engaged in high-effort coping and who live with ongoing, cumulative, and recurrent stress and trauma need. Experiencing safety in stillness supports the ability to calm the nervous system in the face of racial and ethnic wounding. It does not mean you do nothing when action is required, and it's not that the wounds don't hurt—they do. But when you learn to push the pause button before reacting, you avoid being hijacked by fear and anger. You are far less likely to freeze or act out in ways that you will later regret. Instead, you learn to stop. Take a deep breath. Release it. Then let that brief moment of stillness guide you to the best course of action. This is not the stillness of collapse; rather, it is the beginning of wisdom. This is when our responses to ethnic and race-based emotional injury become constructive, creative, and functional.

Restorative Yoga, when practiced regularly, teaches the nervous system what rest and relaxation feel like. When stress and trauma do not remain lodged in the nervous system, you learn to remain non-reactive in stressful situations. Remember, stress is an internal state caused by either an external threat or an internal trigger. The first step in better controlling your body's reaction to external stresses and internal triggers is to practice experiencing calmness in your body. The more you practice what it feels like to be calm, the easier it is to remember the feeling and to call on it in stressful situations. When the nervous system is balanced and the sympathetic and parasympathetic systems are integrated, you can pick up cues of safety in the environment. Then you can be compassionate, curious about the world, and emotionally connected to the people around you.

DO IT SCARED

Many of us associate vulnerability with weakness. But just because you're vulnerable does not make you weak. Reaching out and speaking your truth require stepping into your vulnerability. It is usually not a comfortable feeling and requires strength. We have to fortify ourselves internally so we are not derailed by our emotions when we get triggered by racial insults, or burn out because we're trying so hard to make a difference, or freeze in the face of racially insensitive behaviors that require a response.

This journey is not a safe one. It is a brave one. Disrupting the status quo involves risk. I suppose when you don't know what to say or do, it's better to remain still and silent, but if you're waiting to feel safe before you speak up or stand up, you may never do either. Sometimes we have to be willing to do it scared. Melissa DePino, the woman who shared the coffee-shop video of the two men being arrested, said she had never in her life spoken up or taken action until she did. She did not wait until she felt safe.

It takes awareness, courage, and commitment to speak up, and it helps to have a support system of allies. We need the healing power of relationship. We need to fortify each other. We need to be each other's advocates. That means establishing relationships of mutuality, reciprocity, and trust by showing up safe for one another. This is how we grow together.

REFLECTION

Attuned Relationship: It's Nature's Way

Trees communicate with each other through the scents they emit to attract bees for pollination, to alert other trees to impending danger, and to express care and protection for one another through electrical impulses via their root systems. Attuned relationship is nature's way.

JOSHUA TREES KNOW

Joshua trees know
each other
Root systems connecting
Across vibrational sand
Science says Joshua Trees hum
Sing together
Perhaps amongst their mycelium roots
Or limb to limb
Mystery
Whatever happens to one
Happens to all
Evolved consciousness
Oneness
Joshua trees know
How do we awaken to this too

DISCUSSION

– Has anyone ever been afraid of you because of your ethnicity or race?
– Have you ever been afraid of anyone because of their ethnicity or race?
– When you feel unsafe, what is the story you tell yourself?
– How does the story you create influence the action you take?
– If someone is afraid of you, how do you respond?

- When you are afraid of someone, how do you react? When you feel safe with others, where is that coming from?
- Think about a group of people that you don't want to be around and ask yourself, "What assumptions am I making about those people?"
- Think about a group of people you want to be around and ask yourself, "What assumptions am I making about those people?"

REFERENCES

Benson, H. (1996) *Timeless Healing*. New York, NY: Fireside.

Buczynski, R. and Porges, S. (2012) "Why this Changes Everything." Transcript of a webinar session, Trauma Therapy Series, National Institute for the Clinical Application of Behavioral Medicine. Accessed on 11/14/2019 at www.flexible mindtherapy.com/uploads/6/5/5/2/65520823/nicabm-porges-2012.pdf.

Buczynski, R. and Porges, S. (2015) "Why the Vagal System Holds the Key to the Treatment of Trauma." Transcript of a webinar session, Trauma Therapy Series, National Institute for the Clinical Application of Behavioral Medicine. Accessed on 12/04/2019 at www.soundeducation.com.au/vagal-system-holds-key-treatment-trauma.

Desikachar, T.K.V. (1995) *The Heart of Yoga: Developing a Personal Practice*. Rochester, VT: Inner Traditions International.

Porges, S. (2011) *The Polyvagal Theory*. New York, NY: W.W. Norton & Company.

Chapter 4

ARE YOU IN YOUR SKIN?

WHEN A Peace Corps volunteer arrived in a village in the northern desert of Cameroon, she was anxious to get to work helping the villagers improve their living conditions. She noticed the village women gathered at the water pump laughing and washing clothes, so she joined them. Fluent in the regional language and intent on helping, she expected to be received in a friendly, welcoming way, but no matter how hard she tried to engage with the women, they ignored her. This went on for a period of time before she finally asked another volunteer, who seemed to be accepted, what she should do. The other volunteer taught her a traditional greeting to open conversation with the village women—"Jam bah doo nah?" meaning "Are you in your skin?" Or "Is your soul in your body?" The response to the greeting—"Jam coree doo may"—means, "I am alive and well and in my skin. My soul is in my body." Once the new arrival began to greet them in this way, the village women welcomed her warmly (Herrera 1999). In this context, being in your skin involves an awareness of the connection between your body's state and your soul's primacy. When body, mind, heart, and soul are aligned, they are experienced as one and we feel energized, enlivened, and well.

THE KOSHAS

The aim of yoga is to become aware of the unity of all aspects of your being—your body, mind, and spirit—so that the clear light of the soul shines through your thoughts, emotions, words, actions, and physical body. Yoga philosophy tells us that there are five layers of being called the koshas. Each layer or sheath is interconnected and influences the other. We experience wholeness, health, and well-being when all five sheaths are integrated. The yoga journey guides us from the outermost layer of being, the physical body, to the innermost layer of being, the soul, the core of our being.

When we refer to the body, most of us think of skin, bone, muscle, and internal organs. But our physiology is only one aspect of being. Our outermost layer, the physical body, is called the anamaya kosha and it encompasses the other four aspects of inner being called the subtle body: the pranamaya kosha is the life-force energy that flows through the breath; the manomaya kosha involves the processing of thought and emotion through the thinking mind; the vijnanamaya kosha, or intellect, is awareness that exists beyond the thinking mind and speaks the language of insight, intuition, and wisdom; the anandamaya kosha, the soul or bliss body, is the experience of bliss, not just as feelings of joy, but as our identity. It is a steady state of being, regardless of circumstances. The bliss body is the most refined of the koshas and influences the other four bodies. In contact with this state of being, you experience an integrated sense of wholeness. The bliss body affects all the other koshas, which is why we want to cultivate a relationship with this aspect of our being. As above, so below. As below, so above. As within, so without.

Although many modern-day yogis compare the koshas to Russian nesting dolls that stack in decreasing size one inside the other, or to an onion whose layers are separated by a thin membrane leading to the core, the ancients described our multiple layers of being as clouds that nestle together and merge with each other. Like the clouds that interpenetrate one another, there is no separation between the koshas. When anandamaya, the subtlest layer of being, merges with and dissolves into pure consciousness, we are in direct connection with the divine, the essence of all that is. This is yoga's ultimate goal. You cannot make this happen; you can only engage in practices that support the potential of this occurring. Anandamaya is not a function of the thinking mind. It is a deeper experience that extends beyond thought and language. When the five koshas are aligned, and you are connected to your core, no matter what circumstance arises you are able to maintain a sense of well-being. You are not blinded by emotion or distracted by thoughts. You remain steady, clear, and focused. You are able to maintain your center and avoid acting out even under the most challenging circumstances. When you are out of alignment, your responses to external events are less reliable and you are more likely to react to internal triggers and project them onto external events. Even though our koshas are in play all the time, most of us are only aware of more than one or two at a time. To be fully empowered, you need to tap into the energy of all five of the koshas. This requires an awareness of all five layers of being.

Engaging in a meditation I learned from yoga teacher Eddie Stern is a beautiful way to integrate the koshas in consciousness and to experience and cultivate a relationship with anandamaya kosha.

ANANDAMAYA KOSHA MEDITATION

Come to a seated position with a straight spine either in a chair or on the floor. If on the floor and you need more support, sit with your back supported by a wall behind you. When you are physically comfortable, close your eyes and shift your awareness to your breath. Once you feel settled in, with your eyes still closed, or with lids slightly separated, shift your awareness to your physical body. Systematically, go through each body part from bottom to top, being very specific. Take your time. Focus your awareness on the top of your right foot, then your toes, then the sole of your right foot. Just feel. Then move your attention upward to your ankle, your shin, your calf, your knee, and your thigh. Then move your awareness to the left side and repeat the entire process, starting with the top of your left foot. When you reach your left thigh, move your awareness to your hips, your waist, your torso, your chest, your collarbones, your back, your right shoulder, then your right upper arm, forearm, wrist, hand, and fingers. Next move your awareness to your left fingers, left hand, left forearm, left upper arm, and left shoulder. Now move your awareness to your neck, back, sides, and front, then jaw, ears, cheekbones, eyes, temples, forehead, and scalp. Next turn your focus further inward and direct your awareness to your brain, the inside of your mouth, your esophagus, your lungs, your heart, your diaphragm, your liver, your spleen, your pancreas, your stomach, and your intestines. Once you have completed your external and internal body scan, invite your imagination to envision yourself as a dove. The head of the dove represents joy; the right wing of the dove represents love, the left wing delight. The body of the dove represents bliss and the entire body of the dove is encased in and held by consciousness. Rest in this meditation for as long as you like.

INTEROCEPTION

Interoception is the ability to detect our internal visceral states. It is the ability to know, for example, when you are experiencing pleasure or pain, when you are hungry, thirsty, hot, cold, sleepy, rested, mad, sad, glad, scared, or inspired. Our physical, mental, emotional, and spiritual states of being are connected and constantly interacting. We are capable of monitoring these states and of adapting to meet the need of each state as it arises. Feelings from your body provide you with information about your physical condition and the underlying thoughts, emotional state, and moods that you experience. Your ability to identify, access, understand, and respond appropriately to your internal signals helps you engage with life in ways that allow you to face challenges and make the ongoing adjustments that are necessary and beneficial to your physical, emotional, and spiritual health and well-being.

Our feelings are grounded in the body, not in the mind. To fully appreciate the extent to which the state of your body impacts how you experience life, you have to start paying attention to it. Cultivating interoceptive awareness in the body is a starting point for health, growth, and restoration. We start here because the physical body is the most tangible aspect of being and, though the hardest to change, is the easiest to access. The body registers the pain of ethnic and racial wounding and impacts your thoughts and emotional responses. Even so, it is not uncommon for people who experience the undue stress and trauma of ongoing ethnic and racial wounding to ignore their bodily cues. The ability to ignore or dissociate from ongoing pain is an adaptive strategy. It is passed on from one generation to the next as a way of dealing with the unbearable suffering imposed on black and brown bodies who were/are unable to escape physical abuse, emotional abuse, injustice, the agony of family separation, the fear of bodily harm, and even loss of life. The horrors of the Middle Passage during the Transatlantic Slave Trade, enslavement endured by African people in the Americas and the Caribbean, unjust incarceration, the genocide of Native Americans, the internment of Japanese Americans, and the inhumane detainment of asylum seekers from Central American countries are a few examples. Traumatic injuries endure and strategies for remaining safe get passed down from generation to generation. Over time these reflexive, traumatic responses lose their context, but our bodies still house the unhealed dissonance and trauma of our ancestors and influence our coping strategies (Menakem 2017).

Epigenetic science is now demonstrating that DNA actually changes as these responses to stress and trauma are passed on from one generation to the next. We cannot change the reality of our racial wounds, but we can do something to change our habitual responses and to heal our pain. The yogis tell us that when we heal our own pain, we heal the pain of seven generations behind us and seven generations going forward. When healing occurs, we will not continue to pass on the legacy of denying or hiding racial wounds.

Difficulty arises when adaptive responses to abusive experiences do not change, even when the circumstance has. What at one time may have been a necessary strategy for survival may no longer serve, and may have worse consequences than learning newer, more relevant strategies. Becoming attuned to your physical and emotional pain and suffering, combined with healthy strategies for alleviating distress, is important to growth and development. As part of a self-care strategy, becoming mindfully aware of how stress and trauma register in the body is an important skill to develop. We must make friends with our body. A racing heart, shallow or heavy breathing, a tight jaw, a knotted stomach are signs of distress, but what do they mean? Rhythmic breathing, relaxed facial features, the ability to smile and laugh spontaneously, fluid bodily movement are all signs of well-being. It is important that we respect our body's responses and get curious about what they are, what they mean, when they occur, and what we can do to alleviate distress and enhance well-being.

The physical symptoms of ethnic and racial distress are real. Ignored, misunderstood, and unaddressed, they can manifest as physical illnesses or emotional disturbances that have no apparent cause. It has been determined that in the United States an estimated 60 to 80 percent of medical visits may be due to stress-related issues (Nerurkar *et al.* 2013). Health care providers are not always attuned to ethnic and racial wounding as causes of stress-related illness and can overlook its impact. It was determined that 45 percent of primary care physicians rarely or never discussed stress management with their patients (Avey *et al.* 2003). In order to heal from the wounds of ethnic and race-based stress and trauma you have to know where the emotional states are expressed in your body and how your response to the stress impacts you. Being alert to interoceptive information allows you to be aware of stress-related signals and to respond to the onset of stressful events in a conscious, non-reactive way. The ability to remain non-reactive in the face of a stressful event gives you time to interpret your response and to create a strategy that will support well-being. Sometimes it is as simple as recognizing an internal signal, such as a gripping sensation in your stomach, to know that you have been triggered. With awareness, you can pause, take a deep breath, and let the feeling pass before you take action. Responding in the immediacy of the moment is not always wise.

EMOTIONAL REGULATION

Becoming mindfully aware of where tension is held in your body can help you detect signs of emotional distress before you become overwhelmed, fall ill, or find yourself acting out in ways that may not fit the situation. Angry outbursts or the inability to act when action is required are examples of an overwhelmed nervous system. Awareness of your internal state is an important self-care skill for managing your emotional responses. Your physical bodily sensations communicate to you your emotional state. Tense muscles, a tight jaw, clenched fists, shallow breathing, and rapid heartbeat all communicate stress. When you are attuned to your inner body's cues, you are better able to meet the need being communicated. In the case of the physical cues listed here, the need is to relax and calm down, not to act out. Your emotional responses and your behavior tend to meet your body's needs when you are in touch with the state of your body.

A response that adequately meets the needs of a stressful situation requires emotional regulation. Emotional regulation involves being attuned to cues from your physical body, your subtle body, and the circumstance you find yourself in. It involves calling on behaviors that are growth-enhancing and that optimize well-being. It involves clear, effective communication between all aspects of your being. When your koshas are online and working harmoniously, you are able to tolerate and understand your body's signals and the thoughts and emotions attached to those signals. Your capacity to effectively manage unpleasant sensations and your reactions to them is enhanced. In other words, your ability to detect and then evaluate cues coming from your body in a particular circumstance can lead to behaviors that temper and influence your emotional responses to situations. This is what happened when I was able to tolerate the discomfort of my hair being touched by a yoga teacher long enough to realize that there was no harm intended and no harm done. My ability to remain present and non-reactive in that situation led to healing a long-forgotten race-related wound. Emotional regulation benefits health and well-being, enables us to form and sustain connections with others, and supports the ability to competently manage life's many and varied situations wisely. When wisdom is online, we no longer have to learn by trial and error. Instead, we are able to rely on insight and intuition as our guides. Emotional responses that are out of proportion to the event that triggers the response, or that just don't fit the circumstance, are signs of emotional dysregulation. For example, angry outbursts, the inability to take any action at all, or choosing external solutions to internal problems do nothing to regulate your emotional responses and are not effective for establishing an internal state of well-being. Any good feeling that results is short-lived. Acting out simply reinforces dysregulation and over time leads to anxiety, depression, aggression, and, in the extreme, PTSD. Stress and trauma affect our ability to recognize our internal signals and impair our ability to tolerate discomfort, making it difficult to accurately interpret your body's signals and to make good choices about how to behave in a situation when you are triggered.

Ignoring pain and discomfort does not support emotional regulation. Interoceptive awareness does. What this means is paying attention to your bodily cues helps you understand and interpret the ways stress affects you, and can help you choose behaviors that will adequately meet the need to relieve stress. Learning to pay attention to your inner state of being helps regulate your emotional responses to both minor and major stressors. Knowing where you hold stress in your body and how you are affected mentally and emotionally takes alert awareness and practice.

SAMSKARAS

Yoga philosophy tells us that the Sanskrit word "samskara" explains patterns of behavior that we repeat but that are outside of our conscious awareness. Some samskaras are adaptive and some are maladaptive. Adaptive samskaras reflect virtues that support internal freedom and growth. Kindness, empathy, generosity, and compassion are examples. Maladaptive samskaras are undigested, stored energy that block and inhibit the release of past painful experiences. They manifest as beliefs and behaviors that undermine self-esteem and lead to self-defeating behaviors that hold us hostage and limit growth.

A samskara is a powerful vibrational energy that arises in consciousness after an external event or when an internal trigger stimulates a thought, sensation, or emotion. When it is an emotion that we do not like, or that we cannot handle, we push it out of our awareness. But the emotion does not disappear. Thoughts and emotions are forms of energy, and energy is not created and cannot be destroyed—it can only be transformed. When energy is unbound, it is free to flow without resistance and it releases. Whatever we push out of awareness or cling to because we can't let go becomes blocked energy. It sinks into the subconscious, where it leaves an impression and is stored as a physical and psychological memory. When something internal or external triggers it, the thought, feeling, or emotion returns to the surface level of awareness, looking for an escape route so it can release. If met with resistance again, it returns to the unconscious realm. Over time unreleased energy builds up and spills out in unexpected, unpredictable, and sometimes destructive ways. This is maladaptive. If you don't want to be controlled by your maladaptive samskaras, you have to learn to release the energy blocks they represent. This means crying when you're sad, laughing when you're happy, protesting when you're angry, and seeking safety when you're scared. This is what is meant by letting go and surrendering to reality as it is. This is adaptive.

Blocked energies are stored in the body and the mind and influence your behavior. A maladaptive samskara can also be created when you cling to something that you like. The inability to let go creates a block and leads to pain and suffering when you are unable to re-experience a feeling or sensation that at one time gave you pleasure but no longer does. The attempt to recreate a past experience that you enjoyed is an example. Until you realize that nothing is ever as good as the first time, you keep trying to recreate the original experience. The result is usually frustration and often disillusionment, both painful experiences. Doing the same thing over and over again and expecting a different result is futile.

Samskaras are informed by beliefs, opinions, and assumptions you've absorbed from your family and culture as well as your accumulated mental patterns and your patterns of resistance. These body/mind imprints are considered to be the root of both pleasurable and painful experiences. They have a powerful gravitational pull and cause us to repeat behaviors habitually whether or not we understand why, even if there is no apparent benefit. We are creatures of habit. Each time we repeat an action it creates a stronger imprint and the less inclined we are to choose an action that is contrary to the existing habit. Addictive behaviors are born of samskaras. Shining a light on our repetitive behavior is the first step toward changing old patterns that no longer serve.

What comes to mind is a popular, frequently told, Buddhist parable that illustrates the importance of paying attention to thought patterns and behaviors and releasing them when they do not serve the present moment or the context one finds oneself in.

TWO MONKS CROSSING A STREAM

Two monks, one an elder and one a novice, were traveling together in silence away from the monastery on pilgrimage. As they approached their destination, they had to cross a fast-moving stream. There was no bridge, so they had to find a shallow part of the stream to get safely to the other side. As they searched for the best spot, they came across a young woman standing on the bank of the stream, afraid to cross. The novice, remembering his vows never to touch a woman, nodded as he passed her by, stepped into the stream, and carefully crossed to the other side. Seeing her need, the elder monk picked the frightened woman up and carried her on his back and placed her safely on the far bank of the stream. The woman bowed to the elder monk in gratitude and continued on her way. The novice was disturbed that the elder monk had broken his vow to never touch a woman, and as time went on, he became increasingly angry. Finally, unable to contain himself any longer, he shouted out, "You broke your sacred vow to never touch a woman. How could you do that? You are a disgrace to the monastery." The elder monk, surprised at the outburst, turned to look at the novice and said, "I dropped that woman hours ago. Have you been carrying her all this time?"

When our behavior patterns are habitual and mindless, they lose contextual meaning. We do what we do because that's just the way things are done. There may be a good reason for the behavior in a particular context. In the case of the monks, a vow of celibacy is taken to keep them from being distracted by sexual urges. Out of context—in this instance, helping a terrified woman in need—the vow of celibacy was irrelevant and no longer served a beneficial purpose. This is how samskaras work. They are conditioned responses repetitively done without awareness and out of context. These patterns of behavior are difficult to resist, even when they are no longer beneficial. Our habitual behavior influences our thoughts, the language we use, and the actions we take.

This is where a comprehensive yoga practice that facilitates mental, emotional, and behavioral awareness comes in. The comprehensive path includes the ten ethical principles of living a meaningful, purposeful life, called yamas and niyamas—physical postures of asana, breath practices of pranayama, and meditative practices that help slow the mind, manage emotions, and support psychospiritual development. Comprehensive yoga practices teach us how to allow energy to flow through us as we remain grounded in present-moment awareness. With awareness, we are able to replace maladaptive samskaras with more life-affirming behaviors that support health, growth, and well-being. When we shine the light of awareness on unconscious behaviors, even though our samskaras continue to exist, they no longer have the power to bind us or influence our thoughts and actions. We are able to access the power of discernment and let that guide our actions. Awareness, not denial, is where our freedom lies.

THE PAIN BODY

I was first introduced to the concept of the pain body when I read Eckhart Tolle's book *A New Earth*. He describes the pain body as a kind of life form, an energy that feeds off past emotional pain that has not been fully digested or released (Tolle 2005). On a personal level, think about those times you experience anger, anxiety, depression, or some other unpleasant state that you would rather not. Whether you experience the feeling as strong and overwhelming, or as a mild form of unease, if you find yourself feeding it instead of letting it go, that is the pain body. Once your pain body is activated, it tries to drag anyone close by into its orbit. Misery loves company. Anyone who tries to help you feel better is avoided, verbally attacked, or pushed away. When the pain body takes over, it commandeers your thought process and feeds your emotions with its negative energy. Once it is satisfied, it goes dormant and doesn't resurface until it needs more misery to keep itself going.

The pain body is not only personal; it can be collective as well. The collective pain body is made up of members of tribes, nations, and races who share in the pain body in varying degrees of intensity. Members of racial groups who have suffered persecution over centuries are part of a collective racial pain body (Tolle 2005). Native people and ethnic groups who were the original settlers of a region before invasion and colonization, whose populations were often decimated and cultures co-opted and destroyed, are examples. Another example is the collective pain body of Africans of the diaspora whose ancestors were kidnapped from Africa, dehumanized, beaten into submission, and enslaved throughout the Americas and the Caribbean. The suffering inflicted on these populations becomes part of the collective pain body of entire nations because both perpetrator and victim suffer the consequences of oppression and brutality. Tolle reminds us that because we are all extensions of each other, whatever we do to someone else, we do to ourselves. Resistance to dealing with the pain and suffering caused by ethnic and race-based injury keeps the collective racial pain body alive. It is why nearly all of us, regardless of race or ethnicity, still carry trauma in our bodies around the myth of race.

Some of our emotional pain actually comes from resistance to suffering, the refusal to accept that we are all subject to life's difficulties. Shining the light of awareness on the reality of ethnic and race-based stress and trauma is required to break identification with the pain body. Once that happens, it loses its power. The first noble truth of Buddhism tells us that pain and suffering are a natural part of life, and that once we accept that truth, we will not find it so unbearable. Paradoxically, facing difficulties head on is the beginning of the end of suffering. Yoga tells us that the experience of suffering is often the first step toward positive change. Once something becomes so painful that it disrupts your life, you are more likely to seek a solution. This is universal wisdom. People in 12-step recovery programs know it well.

While relying on the experience of pain and suffering to be your teacher can be an effective way to motivate positive change, we want to grow beyond the experience of pain as our primary teacher and cultivate a relationship with our wisdom body. A willingness to endure pain, both physical and emotional, can be detrimental when it is not balanced with ease and comfort. Restorative Yoga and the contemplative practices of yoga help mitigate the negative impacts of race-based stress and trauma by offering experiences of feeling relaxed, peaceful, and safe in stillness. It is this experience that deepens our sense of well-being.

EMOTIONAL TRIGGERS

Each individual body has its own unique response to stress and trauma, and each body needs and deserves to heal. Identifying our emotional triggers is an important part of the healing process. We experience our triggers physically. They are activated through our sense of sight, sound, touch, smell, and taste. Anything can trigger you depending on your beliefs, values, and earlier life experiences. It can be a request to do something you would rather not do, a tone of voice, a look, someone's appearance, a point of view, an organizational policy, a location; anything that offends, makes you feel small, threatened, stereotyped, invisible, dehumanized, or attacked. Your emotional responses can include fear, anger, hurt, surprise, shame, or embarrassment. When you become triggered emotionally, a cascade of neural, biochemical, and hormonal actions are initiated by the nervous system, causing you to lose present-moment awareness.

Emotional triggers are like invisible landmines. When they are stepped on, they provoke an intense and excessive internal emotional reaction that no one saw coming, not even you. We typically blame our response on the person, event, or circumstance that provoked it, when in fact a trigger is really an experience that brings up the past, causing old feelings and behaviors to arise that you have pushed out of your awareness. It may be hard to believe, but whenever you get triggered, it is actually 90 percent you and only 10 percent the event, circumstance, or the other person that triggered your reaction. This is not to say that there is not an external provocation, but it is to say that your response to whatever provokes you is coming from within you. The way you can tell is that not everyone is responding to sights, sounds, people, places, and events the same way you are. A trigger is something that sets off a memory tape or flashback and transports you back to the event of your original wound or trauma. Owning your responses to what triggers you empowers you to identify and address unhealed stress and trauma. We need to become curious about our triggers.

The goal is not to overcome your triggers, but to recognize a trigger and wait until the feeling passes before you take action. This is emotional regulation. Paradoxically, with practice and over time your emotional triggers will dissolve and your emotional comfort zone will expand.

EMOTIONAL SWEET SPOT

Triggers are deeply personal; different things trigger different people. In the case of a traumatic event, a person may begin to avoid situations and stimuli that they think might trigger a flashback. They fear they might react to a flashback trigger with an emotional intensity similar to the one at the time of their original trauma.

Joyce is a perfect example. She is a dedicated yoga practitioner and gifted yoga teacher with a grasp of yoga philosophy artfully woven into her teachings. Typically calm and even-keeled, under stress Joyce was prone to emotional outbursts that were causing serious problems in her marriage. She came to counseling for help in stabilizing her emotional responses. Even though she knew it would benefit her, Joyce was resistant to cultivating a meditation practice. The thought of being still and "doing nothing" did not make sense to her and frightened her as well. As we explored her resistance, in a moment of candor, she confided that she was terrified of closing her eyes and being still in a meditation or Restorative Yoga practice for fear of having flashbacks to a trauma she experienced as a younger adult. She feared she would break down again as she had done at that time. With gentle and consistent encouragement, over time Joyce agreed to participate in a therapeutic Restorative Yoga class. She was told that she did not have to close her eyes and that at any time she felt unable to remain still she could come out of whatever posture she was in, wait until she felt ready, and then begin again. Participating in a group setting was helpful to her as she did not feel alone and isolated. Remember, being around other settled bodies helps your body settle as well. As she continued the practice, she became less reactive, her moods began to stabilize, and her marriage improved. Gradually, and over a period of time, she became dedicated to her Restorative Yoga practice and decided to try meditation. Again she was instructed to meditate with a downward gaze rather than with closed eyes. She did this until she felt comfortable meditating with her eyes closed. As her overall sense of well-being improved, she incorporated meditation into her daily routine, and now practices for 20 minutes twice daily. She has even begun to teach meditation.

Each of us has a psychological, physiological, and behavioral comfort zone. In your comfort zone you feel cool, calm, collected, and safe. You are able to control your emotional state, handle people and relationship challenges, and soothe yourself when you get triggered. Outside your comfort zone you may feel on edge, unsettled, anxious, angry, or unsafe. We each have different bandwidths of comfort. The comfort zone is that space between hyper-arousal and hypo-arousal. Some of us can be catapulted outside of our comfort zone by a seemingly insignificant occurrence, while others seem unfazed by a catastrophic event. It all depends on the range of your comfort zone.

In an active asana practice we encourage yoga practitioners to approach their physical body with awareness to prevent injury. Breath is the focal point. When breathing becomes labored, we are working too hard. When it is shallow, we are not engaged enough. In a Restorative Yoga practice we want to support practitioners in approaching their psychological and emotional body, their subtle energy body, without triggering a state of hyper- or hypo-arousal. We follow the Goldilocks principle of not too cold, not too hot, but just right. We utilize breath by extending the exhale to be twice as long as the inhale to calm the nervous system. If more stimulation is needed, we emphasize a longer inhale. When a state of homeostasis is reached, inhale and exhale are equal in length. In an active physical practice we caution those who are hyper-flexible not to stretch too far, to prevent injury. We remind those who have a limited range of motion that over time, by honoring their physical limitations, they will develop a greater range of motion. It is through the process of awareness that we learn our optimal physical range at any given time. The same is true of our psychological range of motion. Just because we can tolerate stress does not mean we should ignore the signals that tell us we have either gone too far or not far enough.

When we feel anxious, overwhelmed, have emotional outbursts, become aggressive, or when we shut down, become depressed, forgetful, and not present, we have exceeded our capacity for emotional stimulation and are no longer in our sweet spot. Behaviorally, when we become rigid, obsessive, or compulsive in our thoughts and behavior, impulsive in our actions, or disconnected, emotionless, and operating on autopilot, we have exceeded our limit. As we become familiar with our emotional tolerance for resting in stillness and honor it, over time and bit by bit, like Joyce, our safe zone expands and we can meet being still with less reactivity. Our safe zone can be broadened through experiences of safety in stillness. Growth occurs when we are able to stretch into new places without becoming overwhelmed. Self-exploration through the practice of Restorative Yoga enhances awareness of our physiological states of stress and relaxation. Our ability to understand our body's responses to environmental cues aids in developing emotional regulation. The more able we are to tolerate our physiological responses, the more likely we are to expand our emotional sweet spot between being hyper-aroused and hypo-aroused. Expanding the sweet spot is not for the purpose of adapting to oppressive or racist situations. Its purpose is to reduce reactivity, so that we are able to work toward effectively managing and even changing an oppressive situation. By maintaining attention to present-moment awareness with an attitude of openness, curiosity, and self-compassion, Restorative Yoga supports interoceptive awareness and emotional regulation incrementally in a safe and conscious manner. Body awareness and emotional regulation go hand in hand. Yoga offers both.

BODY, MIND, HEART, AND SOUL IN HARMONY

At a personal growth workshop conducted for men, in a discussion on challenges they face in their places of employment, Marcus, one of the participants, who prior to becoming a student of Restorative Yoga had a history of losing his temper when provoked, told the following story:

One day, he overheard one of his co-workers say in reference to a problem that needed to be resolved, "Let the 'n – – – er' fix it." Being the only African American in the room, just to make sure he heard what he thought he did, he asked the man to repeat himself. So the man repeated it. Instead of blowing up or getting into a physical altercation as he would have in the past, Marcus said a feeling of calm came over him. He finished his shift and went to his supervisor and told him what happened. The supervisor agreed that the comment was completely out of order and asked Marcus how he wanted the situation handled. Marcus thought for a moment and said, "I don't want him to lose his job because I realize that could have been me several years ago when I used to blow up at the drop of a hat. But I want him held to account for what he said because it was hurtful. I think he should be suspended." The offending man was suspended for two days without pay. The other men in the workshop, hearing the story, reacted by telling Marcus, "You let him get away with that? You should have taken legal action." "I wish somebody would call me that. After I kicked his butt, I'd sue first and then get him fired." They reacted with feelings of anger and confused Marcus's measured response with passivity and weakness. They didn't know his history of angry outbursts, and did not know that years of therapy and a consistent Restorative Yoga practice enabled him to remain calm enough not to act out in the situation. Marcus was not derailed by his feelings and was able to respond compassionately.

When body, mind, heart, and soul are aligned, we are guided by insight, wisdom, and clarity, not by emotion. Our practices support us in remaining open to our feelings, and instead of pushing an experience beneath conscious awareness because it hurt, or acting out because we are triggered, we allow ourselves to be impacted by the experience, but not hijacked by it. There is a difference. You are neither suppressing nor expressing when your body, mind, heart, and soul are in harmony with the reality of an external situation. You are experiencing the upward flow of unblocked emotional energy that can move through you. And the downward flow of unblocked spiritual energy from the anandamaya kosha that nourishes you. When all of our koshas are in harmony, we experience well-being and wholeness regardless of the situation or circumstance we find ourselves in. It does not mean that we don't feel hurt, sad, mad, glad, or scared. We do. It means that when we are aligned, we are able to experience the full range of human emotion in harmony with whatever life presents. Harmony is the moment-to-moment exchange of what's happening internally and externally. Things are going to happen in life that will hit you hard and that you are unable to change or control. When we are unable to change the circumstance causing our suffering, and instead surrender to reality as it is, paradoxically we move beyond suffering and come to a place of peaceful acceptance. It is from this place that we are able to see with more clarity. If action is required, we can be creative, instead of reactive, and make the best choice.

A consistent practice of Restorative Yoga and meditation helps us embody this reality, eventually making calm, compassionate, wise responses our default. There is an old Zen saying that can help guide our healing practice. It tells us that when we are no longer offended by what has previously been an emotional trigger, the thing no longer exists. Resting in awareness of our true self helps us reach this state of being.

REFLECTION

Soulful Living

Each of us has a need to belong, to feel as though we are part of a community. We long for connection with others. It's the most natural thing in the world. Being an outsider can cause us to feel the pain of alienation, so we sometimes sacrifice our aloneness to be with others, trying to fit in, even when we are not welcomed. Although the circumstances vary, each of us at various times in our lives has had to confront our sense of isolation. As painful and scary as it can be, experiencing your aloneness can teach you how to enjoy the pleasure of your own company and how to welcome and fit in with yourself. Learning to welcome and fit in with yourself and welcoming and fitting in with others are complementary. They go hand in hand.

Embracing aloneness teaches you how to sit through the discomfort of loneliness so you can get to the other side of it and realize it did no harm. Embracing aloneness teaches you how to be in your own skin and prepares you for being in healthy relationships with others. Sitting with our aloneness requires courage and begs the question "How do I live in my own skin? How do I live with myself as an autonomous being?" Loneliness is the soul's longing for itself and should not be avoided. It is a sign of spiritual hunger pangs. It is the longing for connection not just to others; it is an invitation to come home to self. Learning to cherish and enjoy your solitude rather than fearing and avoiding it allows you to actively begin to know and like yourself. It gives you time to think about how you want to be treated by others and time to practice treating yourself the way you want others to treat you.

Loneliness is not meant to be endured as a state of being, but periods of aloneness are required for times of reflection and rejuvenation. It is a stop along the way to becoming your own best friend, and to enjoying the pleasure of your own company. That is our work as evolving human beings. In order to create optimal relationships with others, we have to create optimal relationships with our self. How? Get to know yourself. Learn to love yourself. Spend time alone with yourself. Periods of aloneness offer the opportunity to step more fully into yourself, into your soul. To be able to enjoy aloneness, we need to learn to embrace loneliness when it visits us, like a welcomed guest, to go deep inside of it, and make friends with it, not turn away from it.

When we miss the company of a friend, we reach out. We don't hesitate to call, text, email, or visit. So the next time you feel lonely, before you distract yourself by seeking the companionship of someone else, eating another cupcake, going shopping and spending money you don't have, turning on the TV, or reaching for another glass of wine, put in a call to your soul. Instead of reaching out, reach in and ask yourself, "Am I in my skin? Is my soul in my body?" Sit in your aloneness until the answer is "Yes, I am alive and well and in my skin. My soul is in my body." And when that answer comes, you know you have come home to the most important company you will ever keep—yourself. This is the art of soulful living.

DISCUSSION

Take some time to think about what triggers you and then identify how your body reacts.

When I am triggered:

- my heart beats faster
- my breathing is shallow
- I breathe faster
- my chest feel tight
- I freeze
- my stomach aches
- my head throbs
- I yell
- I lose my voice
- my shoulders get tight
- my back goes out
- my throat closes up
- I cry
- I laugh out loud
- my legs feel heavy
- my arms feel heavy
- I feel flushed and hot
- I feel clammy and cold.

REFERENCES

Avey, H., Matheny, K.B., Robbins, A., and Jacobson, T.A. (2003) "Health care providers' training, perceptions, and practices regarding stress and health outcomes." *Journal of the National Medical Association 95*, 9, 833, 836–845.

Herrera, S. (1999) *Mango Elephants in the Sun: How Life in an African Village Let Me Be in My Skin*. Boston, MA: Shambhala Publications.

Menakem, R. (2017) *My Grandmother's Hands: Racialized Trauma and the Mending of Our Bodies and Hearts*. Las Vegas, NV: Central Recovery Press.

Nerurkar, A., Bitton, A., Davis, R., Phillips, R.S., and Yeh, G. (2013) "When physicians counsel about stress: Results of a national study." *JAMA Internal Medicine 173*, 1, 76–77.

Tolle, E. (2005) *A New Earth: Create a Better Life*. New York, NY: Penguin Books.

Chapter 5

SHINE A LIGHT

I MET a White South African at a yoga conference who, in a conversation about race and ethnicity, shared how surprised he was when he discovered his internalized racial bias. He grew up during the apartheid era, raised by parents who abhorred the system and taught him to abhor it too. He said he didn't discover how indoctrinated and conditioned by the system he was until he came to the United States. In South Africa during the apartheid era, Native (Blacks), Indian, and Colored (Mixed Race) people understood their status as being subordinate to Whites and were expected to defer to them. When non-White people in the United States acted as if they were his equal, he was shocked to discover that he was offended. All of us are the products of our cultural conditioning. It shapes our perceptions of what is safe and what is dangerous, who is superior and who is inferior, who is entitled and who is not, and what is race-based and what is not. None of us is immune from inheriting the biases, stereotypes, and blind spots of our society, no matter how enlightened we may think we are.

Sometimes we have to be removed from our culture of origin to realize how profoundly it has shaped us. Or we can engage in conversation with others, engage in self-reflection, and shine a light on our own ethnic, racial, and cultural blind spots. Because of our blind spots we don't always recognize what we see for what it is. Michelle Saahene called attention to the coffee-shop arrest, mentioned earlier in the book, as being racially motivated as soon as she saw what was happening. Even though no one else seemed to notice until she pointed it out, it was clear to her that the young men who were arrested were being racially profiled. She said later, in an interview about the incident, "We see racism, we just don't acknowledge its existence." Melissa DePino's response to Michelle's calling attention to what was happening was to join her in speaking up. She then tweeted a video of the incident and it went viral. Her tweet said, "All the other white ppl are wondering why it's never happened to us when we do the same thing." Why? Because it's the shadow side of racialized cultures. Unless and until we shine a light on our shadow, there is no possibility of change. It is important that we start paying attention to the effect racializing has on members of racially subordinated groups, and on racially dominant groups too. Let's not be blind to our own cultural conditioning.

ME AND MY SHADOW

Our shadow is the part of us that we do not see or recognize. When we continue to avoid it, because we are uncomfortable with the feelings that arise in us when we see it, it doesn't go away. It just grows larger, takes on a life of its own, pops up to embarrass us, and keeps us from growing. The Eurocentric perspective of shadow would have you believe that your shadow side is your dark side, and darkness in the Eurocentric consciousness is associated with danger, foreboding, and negativity— something to fear. But there are other ways to view shadow. Children run from them, chase them, play hide and go seek with them, and project images onto walls to make art with them. A shadow has shape, color, texture, and mass; it is tangible. To a child, a shadow is a cherished friend. In Navajo culture the shadow is regarded as a sacred part of the self, part of one's spiritual identity. It is not considered a deficient aspect of self that needs to be corrected and returned to a state of wholeness. It is the recognition that as a spiritual being one is already whole. And as a physical being there is no imperfection. It is described as "the dynamic portal from which you are observed by the world of spirit" (West 2018, paragraph 2). African American psychologist, yogi, and scholar Edward Bruce Bynum tells us that "wisdom sleeps behind our psychological fear of the darkness" (Bynum 2012, p.13). So from this perspective shadow hides wisdom. Cut off from wisdom, we remain immature.

As an example, the story of Peter Pan, the boy who never grew up, comes to mind. The story begins when Peter loses his shadow. He returns to the place he lost it to reattach it to his body. As I see it, in order to grow up we have to find and reattach our shadow self, which is our unexamined self. This is not necessarily our so-called bad self. For many descendants of formerly enslaved people in the United States, for instance, hiding or downplaying excellence was an adaptive strategy for fear of being punished for outshining those who, in order to feel good about themselves, need to feel superior. To this day, demonstrations of excellence are a threat to the status quo of racial superiority dating all the way back to laws that prohibited enslaved people in the United States from learning to read and write or from trying to advance themselves in any way.

By the time we reach adulthood, many of us have been conditioned to fear the shadow side of life. Because the shadow represents our unacknowledged traits and unknown characteristics, we refer to it as our dark side. Fearing what we may encounter if we step into our darkness— our unknown, unclaimed self—many of us prefer to avoid it. It scares us because we think of it as something separate and apart from us. Instead of playing hide and go seek as we did as children, we hide from our shadow and it hides from us. But when you find the courage to look for it, to stare it in the face, and step deep into its darkness, you can discover buried treasure. Your shadow holds within it your untapped potential.

The traits that you learn to regard as bad, shameful, or wrong move into your shadow space, where you lose touch with those parts of yourself. Embracing your shadow helps you to see yourself more clearly. Instead of feeling ashamed, you feel compassionate; instead of feeling embarrassed, you feel courageous; instead of feeling limited, you experience freedom. Embracing your shadow allows you to be whole, to be real, to be powerful, to express your passion, and to make your dreams a reality. Your authentic self is acceptable because you are complete, not because you are good. Do not hide from your shadow. Shine the light of awareness on your darkness. When you label yourself as bad, wrong, inferior, or unworthy, you are looking through a distorted lens. Turn your gaze inward and you will become aware that you are complete and whole at the deepest level. The more you are aware, the more you will accept yourself. All parts of you deserve to be seen, heard, and embraced. Every part of you holds a gift that deserves healthy expression. Bringing light to your darkness will support you in creating loving relationships, good emotional health, and achieving your potential. The journey to wholeness requires that we take a look at the best in us, not just the worst in us. It invites us to stop hiding from ourselves. It allows us to know the freedom of living not a perfect life but a transparent life.

Examining the shadow does not have to be a frightening process. What we are trying to do here is to recognize the effect racializing has on those who are racialized, those who do the racializing, and those who deny the existence of racializing. Whether you like it or not, we live in a racialized culture. In racialized cultures, when we forego noticing race, we are unable to engage in adult discourse about the harmful effects that come from ignoring this aspect of one's identity. It becomes the elephant in the room. Let's approach our shadow with curiosity, not dread. In this exploration, two questions emerge. Are you willing to see the process of racializing in others? Are you willing to see it in yourself?

CULTURAL CONDITIONING

So far we have reviewed what ethnic and race-based stress and trauma is, and how it differs from PTSD. We have reviewed how the nervous system works automatically to identify safety and danger and how our nervous system responds to these cues, and we have reviewed how stress and trauma land in our bodies. In this chapter we will review how our cultural conditioning shapes our perceptions of what is safe and what is dangerous, what is race-based and what is not. We have cultural identities and individual identities, and we have group identities too. Whether or not we admit it, each of us is part of a racial and ethnic group identity. There are many categories of identity and in this chapter we will explore how cultural conditioning, dominant racial group identities, and subordinated racial group identities influence and shape consciousness, and how our conditioning can cloud our perceptions. And we will discuss how yoga can help lift the veil, enhance clarity, and support harmony.

The way we gather and process information is culturally determined. Western cultures tend to rely on data-driven, evidence-based, objective information that is devoid of emotional content. In the West this is called objectivity and is regarded as the most valid way to present and process information. But is it really?

MENTAL HEALTH

Approaches to supporting mental health and well-being are not universal but are influenced by culture. Writer Andrew Solomon was curious about various ways different cultures dealt with depression, so he went on a search to find out. He shared a story about a conversation he had with a Rwandan about how they treated depression after the genocide of 1994. The story has been shared on various websites and can be found in numerous blog posts, but Solomon originally shared the story in a 2013 TED Talk (Solomon 2013). Solomon learned that the prescription for depression the Rwandans used was a combination of sun, drum, dance, and community. He learned that when Western mental health workers arrived after the genocide to help the survivors recover, the Rwandans had to ask some of them to leave. The Western mental health approach to healing was to take people individually into what was described as a dingy little room and have them talk about the bad things the survivors had experienced. In Rwandan culture this was considered to be a destructive approach. The Rwandan approach to healing trauma and depression involved a ritual that included the entire community. Everyone would take the day off to be outdoors in the sun, with drummers and people dancing together to get the life force flowing, to lift each other up, and to return one another to joy. To them, depression was regarded as something invasive and external that could be cast out, not something internal that needed to be cured.

PERSONAL GROOMING

In 2019 the state of California banned discrimination against students and employees who wear natural hairstyles. This law had to be instituted because a standard of beauty that is uniformly applied in Western culture does not apply to girls and women with kinky hair. In the United States, unless your hair is straight, wearing your hair the way it naturally grows out of your head is banned altogether or, if your texturized hair does not conform to the cultural standard of straight hair, you are subjected to unequal treatment in work environments and humiliation from the dominant culture (Bates 2017). This does not just apply to women. Think about the way the high school wrestler was humiliated publicly when the wrestling referee forced him to cut off his dreadlocks under threat of forfeiting his entire team's match, rather than just allowing him to cover his hair. The California law called the CROWN Act was actually inspired by this incident. The Governor of the state observed that forcing the student to cut his hair was the same as asking him to choose whether to "lose an athletic competition or lose his identity" (Willon and Díaz 2019, paragraph 2).

In the United States, schools, workplaces, and public venues that are biased toward straight hair are not traditionally safe havens for those with naturally kinky hair on display. As recently as 2017, some school districts in the United States banned girls with kinky hair from wearing braid extensions, afros, dreadlocks, cornrows, and twists, claiming they were distracting, messy, and unkempt. A study was conducted called "The Good Hair Study" (Martin 2017). The results of the study concluded that of the 4000 participants, regardless of race and gender, most people in the study favored straight hair as the accepted standard of beauty. It also found that in attempts to meet the Western standard of what is considered aesthetically pleasing, women with texturized hair suffer more anxiety and spend more money around hair issues than women with straight hair. According to the study, women with texturized hair are subject to unequal treatment in work environments and are viewed as inferior. Women with naturally kinky hair, in this kind of cultural environment, are sensitive about their hair texture for good reason.

ACCULTURATION IS WOUNDING

The process of acculturation is another psychological and physiological risk factor for people. Acculturation is the adoption of dominant cultural values, beliefs, and behaviors, and adapting to cultural norms and physical characteristics you may not share. For example, blending into the dominant culture is required to be regarded as a "true" American. In the case of immigrant populations, learning not to speak your language of origin in public spaces and masking an accent for fear of being shamed or bullied are just two examples. Some children are even sent to speech therapy to rid them of accented speech. Acculturation is not limited to immigrants coming to the United States from other countries. People of various ethnicities and cultures born and raised in the United States, who do not have white skin or resemble people of European ancestry, are continually having to adjust to norms that do not reflect their racial, ethnic, or cultural identity. There are psychological (depression and anxiety) and physiological (diabetes and obesity) consequences of ethnic and racial trauma involved in the process of acculturation because it is stressful (Liu *et al.* 2019). Acculturation involves dressing in a particular way, wearing your hair in a particular way, speaking in a particular way, having light-colored skin, and adopting behaviors and attitudes that soften your racial, ethnic, or cultural presence. This begins early in childhood and continues throughout one's adult life. Acculturation is not a one-time-only process. It is ongoing and continuous. Giving up your identity to fit in is stressful and wounding, and requires ongoing self-care strategies that support resilience, health, and well-being.

BARRIERS TO UNDERSTANDING

All racial, ethnic, and cultural identities are not created equal. Unexamined cultural conditioning can create barriers to understanding each other, causing misapprehension and disharmony between people. Not acknowledging this causes harm. To overcome barriers to understanding, we first have to ground ourselves in the awareness of our membership as part of a racial collective. First, we start with the awareness that we are all members of the human race. But because we live in a racialized culture, depending on your ethnic and racial group identity, you are having experiences that are unique and different from those with different ethnic and racial group identities. When you don't understand this, you can negate someone else's experience by assuming they see events through your lens, and by trying to get them to agree with your perspective. Assuming that we are all having the same experience, coupled with the need for agreement and sameness, leads to misunderstanding and disagreement. Recognizing that your experience and context is unique to you and to the racial or ethnic group to which you belong is key. Listening to a perspective that is different from yours, and trying to understand it, whether you agree with it nor not, is the path toward attuned connection.

Trying to get someone to agree with your perspective is never helpful and can devolve into arguments. What if, rather than trying to get agreement from others, we decided to get to know each other instead? For this to happen we have to be willing to engage with them and listen. Each of us wants to be heard. When we feel unheard or misunderstood, we shout. But shouting just creates more distance between us. It turns us off and we retreat into our own internal place of safety. We shut down. Remember, when our nervous system picks up cues of danger, we stop listening. Shouting does not make anyone feel safe. What if, instead of shouting to be heard, we used our social engagement features? What if we maintained eye contact, listened to the other person, maintained present-moment awareness, and spoke in soothing tones of voice? How might that change our interactions with each other?

Harmonious relationships require awareness, not agreement. The search for agreement leads to arguments because it invalidates the other person's perspective, whereas the search for understanding dissolves the barriers that result in discord and harm, and allows us to get to know one another. In racialized cultures, understanding the profile of racially dominant and racially subordinated group dynamics is an important step on the path to understanding ourselves and each other, and to supporting attuned connection. It starts by recognizing cultural and racial group dynamics.

CULTURAL GROUP DYNAMICS

When my son was in the eighth grade, his piano teacher entered him into a competition that took place at a local university. Since this particular competition favored classical piano pieces, the teacher wanted him to play the *Warsaw Concerto*. The Merriam-Webster Dictionary defines "classical" as "of, relating to, or being music in the educated European tradition that includes such forms as art, song, chamber music, opera, and symphony as distinguished from folk or popular music or jazz" (Merriam-Webster 2019). My son could play the *Warsaw Concerto* but didn't like it. He insisted on playing Stevie Wonder's classic "Ribbon in the Sky," instead. All of the other students who entered into the competition, most of whom were African American, played what would be called traditional European classical pieces. Some of the students' performances were quite impressive. When it was my son's turn to play, he performed "Ribbon in the Sky." You could have heard a pin drop in the auditorium, and when he finished, after a short pause, the audience erupted into applause and gave him a standing ovation. He didn't win the competition and was not awarded second or third place either. His teacher explained that even though my son's rendition was flawless, soulful, and heartfelt, it was not classical. The message that was communicated, whether intended or not, was your piece was good, but not good enough because it did not fit the European standard of what classical is. In this instance the dominant group culture determined what was regarded as classical music and what was not. My son was perplexed but not deterred. He knew he had done a good job. To a twelve-year-old, whose culture regarded jazz, R&B, and hip-hop as classical, the explanation didn't make much sense. Fortunately, my son didn't personalize this experience or internalize it as evidence that he was not good enough. He was grounded in his racial group identity and in the norms of his culture, and was able to get over his disappointment relatively easily. He insisted that he knew he had performed well, was glad he chose "Ribbon in the Sky," and still did not like the *Warsaw Concerto*. He didn't win the competition that day, but he won something much more valuable: a sense of self-efficacy and self-determination.

RACIAL GROUP STATUS

Racial group dominance is the power to influence and normalize preferences and prejudices, what is acceptable and unacceptable, and which ethnic, racial, and cultural groups have status and which do not. Dominant racial group status carries with it the power to impose standards of behavior and establish norms that can ignore and infringe on the rights, customs, values, beliefs, and thought processes of those belonging to racially subordinated groups. Dominant group status has nothing to do with being in the majority. Think South African apartheid. South African Whites were in the clear minority—only 13 percent compared with a 76 percent Native (Black) majority—yet they had the power to create laws and impose standards of behavior that infringed on the rights and jeopardized the safety, health, and well-being of those in the majority.

Typically, members of dominant racial groups do not identify themselves as members of a racial group, but instead see themselves as individuals, and attribute their success and good fortune to their individual efforts. Racial group dominance has nothing to do with how you behave individually or how you are perceived individually, and has more to do with the inherent power and advantages associated with the dominant culture. If you do not identify yourself as a member of a racial group, this can be difficult to comprehend, but recognizing the impact of dominant group power to set social norms that can either do harm or promote justice, equal opportunity, safety, health, and well-being for all people, regardless of race or ethnicity, matters. You may not think it matters if you are not personally negatively impacted or disadvantaged by various established societal norms, but it matters because what impacts one of us impacts all of us, and each individual has a role to play.

The characteristics of subordinated racial group dynamics are different from dominant racial group dynamics. Rather than establishing social norms, people in subordinated racial groups are expected to conform to established social norms and become more like the dominant racial group. Even though becoming more like the dominant group is rewarded to some extent, those in subordinated groups suffer for giving up aspects of who they are to become more like the dominant group. Giving up one's identity to become more like those in the dominant group has destructive consequences to overall health and well-being. Not regarded as individuals, members of subordinated groups are lumped into group identities categorized as minorities, underserved, underprivileged, at risk, or, most recently, as people of color, implying otherness, inferior status, and negating individual identity. Over time, if internalized, these labels can undermine feelings of self-worth and create a sense of invisibility. Subordinated group members want to be acknowledged, validated, and accepted for who they are, not as being a stereotype, as an exception to a stereotype, or as a group.

Racial distress and suffering have united members of subordinated groups, and when harm comes to anyone associated with subordinated group status, they feel the pain as if it were their own. Like the damaging effects of secondhand smoke, secondary or vicarious stress and trauma from observing harm toward others with whom you identify can be devastating.

The differences in life experience based on ethnic and racial group status are real. If we are to engage with one another across our various racial group identities and build bridges toward understanding, we must be willing to acknowledge that our racial and cultural group identities influence our assumptions and our biases, and will incline us toward certain ways of perceiving reality and disincline us toward other ways of perceiving. If we are oblivious to our cultural conditioning and the biases and assumptions that such conditioning holds, we live in a state of ignorance, remain in the dark, and are bound to make mistakes that do harm to ourselves and to others.

CULTURAL BLIND SPOTS

Perceptions of race, ethnicity, and skin color matter, and have an impact on all of us, not just some of us. The dominant cultural group norm is to avoid mentioning, to deny noticing any difference between races and ethnicities, or to become defensive, to behave indignantly, and to take a superior stance if the topic comes up. Unless the intention is to support the racial hierarchy that already exists, this conditioning is not relevant within a multiracial, multiethnic culture. As the yoga community becomes more racially and ethnically varied, if we want to remain relevant, it is in everyone's best interest to examine outdated cultural paradigms and consider replacing them with new ones that better serve a racially and ethnically diverse culture.

But what are our blind spots and how do we know where they are if we can't see them? You have to look for them. When my father, who was a professional pilot, taught me how to drive, he taught me that looking straight ahead was not good enough, that avoiding blind spots required looking through the rear- and side-view mirrors as well as seeing what was in front of me. The same is true of our cultural blind spots. To see them, looking straight ahead is not enough. We have to look around and we also have to look within. Our cultural blind spots might be called our cultural kleshas, those things that we are unable to see. Knowing they are there helps us navigate more clearly. If you are unaware, you are more vulnerable to colliding with the objects you don't see coming your way. Finding our blind spots can help to avoid such collisions.

CULTURE OF SILENCE

We live in a culture of silence regarding race, ethnicity, and skin color. The belief of the dominant cultural group has been, and for many continues to be, that talking about race is racist and divisive. But in a racially and ethnically diverse world, it is time to challenge the cultural norm of silence regarding ethnic, racial, and cultural differences. Conversation is a healing balm that helps us form attuned relationships. It might be uncomfortable, even painful at first, but as we become more adept through practice, the discomfort eases and the wounds of separation begin to heal. Conversation does not divide us; silence does. But it takes willingness, courage, skill, and fortitude to engage in this dialogue. If we don't make it our business to engage in important and constructive conversations about race and ethnicity, we remain trapped in culturally conditioned responses that stunt our personal and spiritual growth. Listening is an important part of the conversation.

During the Civil Rights movement, the chief law enforcement officer of the United States, Bobby Kennedy, invited high-profile Civil Rights activists to meet with him to fill him in on what was happening in the movement. Among those invited were James Baldwin, Harry Belafonte, Lena Horne, and playwright Lorraine Hansberry. The invited guests thought they were called to the meeting to share how devastating poverty and the barriers to equality, access, and success under Jim Crow laws were causing unbearable suffering to African Americans. They assumed it would be an opportunity to express what they thought the Kennedy administration ought to be doing about it. Bobby Kennedy had a different agenda. His intention was to use the meeting as a chance to share all the things he and his brother, President John Kennedy, were doing to try to improve conditions. He expected that their efforts would be acknowledged and applauded by his guests. He was surprised to be greeted with frustration, and criticism from those in attendance who were upset about what the Kennedy administration was failing to do. The meeting was described as heated. Everyone was angry, including Kennedy, and the meeting ended on a note of discord. But then something happened. Kennedy, who was known as a self-reflective man, was able to put himself in the shoes of the people who had approached him with such passion, and decided that they were right, and that he would do something about it. He decided to visit the aggrieved communities and observe firsthand the suffering people endured so he could understand. (Based on Bates 2018)

Kennedy listened, he heard, and he was changed by what he heard. Deep listening has a way of doing that. It involves listening not from the mind, but from the heart. It is an important part of conversation, but sometimes requires sitting in the fire of our own discomfort to do so. This is where the practice of being still and non-reactive is helpful. It helps us get our internal triggers under control by inviting self-reflection before we act. We already know that acting out when we are triggered is not a good idea.

COLOR BLINDNESS

Skin color matters. We are a visual species who respond to each other's appearance, and we attach meaning to skin color. There is a skin-color hierarchy in many cultures that is established by the dominant group. Claiming to be as tan or darker than people in non-White racial groups does not change that. In the United States, differences in skin color were used as a tool to dehumanize, enslave, and oppress Africans, to decimate

Native American populations, and to elevate European colonists. A social hierarchy developed that placed Whites at the top, Blacks at the bottom and other non-Whites somewhere in between. This color hierarchy became the norm and is persistent and wounding. We currently see it in immigration policies designed to exclude people from Middle Eastern, Caribbean, and Latin American countries, to keep them from gaining access to asylum and/or full citizenship opportunities in the United States. Skin-color hierarchy was also established in India during British colonization. Fairer-skinned Indians were afforded economic, educational, and political opportunities that darker-skinned Indians were not. The irony here is that Kali, one of the most revered goddesses in the Hindu pantheon of deities, is depicted as black. She is called the primordial mother whose blackness absorbs all colors.

We deny or ignore skin-color hierarchy at our own peril and the peril of others. The manager of the coffee shop who falsely accused the two men who were arrested of wrongdoing apparently did not recognize her culturally conditioned response for what it was, and mishandled her discomfort by calling the police. This was an action that not only endangered others but cost her her job.

Claiming not to see skin color is a false claim. To illustrate that point, in a presentation I made to yoga therapists called "White Is a Color Too," I asked the 95 percent White audience to look at the back of their hand and identify what color it was. The melanated people in the audience had no trouble identifying what color they saw. Even though most White people in the audience had never done it before, they too, with some difficulty at first, were all able to attach a color to their skin tone. The claim that "I don't see skin color" is a defense against being considered racist. But the claim of color blindness actually helps maintain the status quo of racial superiority and inferiority. Denying that one sees skin color implies that those who do see skin color are in some way inferior to those who do not. The cultural norm of color blindness needs to be challenged. In a racialized culture, race and skin color have meaning and to dismiss both as meaningless is harmful. All of us need to become conscious of the skin-color hierarchy imposed by the dominant group and ask who benefits most? And how can I use my dominant group advantage or skin-color advantage to advocate for and support others?

WHITE PRIVILEGE

In the 1960s segregation was declared illegal and affirmative action became the law of the land. During this period in American history, the term "White privilege" was used to educate dominant group members about the protections and advantages they were afforded by custom and by law, which they had not previously recognized as privileges, and which benefited them solely on the basis of the skin-color hierarchy established in the United States—the right to vote, the right to citizenship, the right to own property, for example. The term "White privilege" was used to explain that subordinated racial groups were not granted the same skin-color opportunities, privileges, and protections, and were penalized because of dark skin. The concept of White privilege was used to stress to the dominant group the necessity of desegregation and affirmative action laws to level the playing field, to equalize protections under the law, and to equalize educational and economic opportunities for all citizens of the United States.

In the twenty-first century, the term "White privilege" has taken on different meanings. It is sometimes declared as proof of "wokeness," and worn either as a badge of honor or as a source of shame. At other times it is used as an explanation, apology, or excuse for being unaware. The term has become a trope. When used as proof of "wokeness," or shame, either way, the term becomes a form of self-aggrandizement. It is enough for one to be aware that there are skin-color privileges associated with light skin without having to announce one's awareness of it by using the term as a descriptor to demonstrate one's "awakeness." When used as an apology or an excuse to explain a lack of awareness, or to explain the failure to take appropriate action when necessary, it suggests that ignoring skin-color hierarchy is merely a mistake, and not a choice. It implies that retreating into claims of White privilege should be a sufficient explanation for a lack of awareness, oblivion, or ignorance. In the twenty-first century it is no longer enough to make the claim of White privilege as a sign of being awake, or to use it as an excuse. It would seem, if one is truly awake or trying to be, that claiming ignorance of and oblivion to what is going on in the global and racialized cultures in which one lives should not be attributed to privilege but should be attributed to the choices one is making to live an insulated life and to ignore certain realities.

These observations may sound harsh, but sometimes wake-up calls sound that way, and this is a wake-up call. The language we use matters.

Asserting White privilege as proof of being awake, or as an apology, explanation, or excuse for a lack of knowledge or awareness, is not an informed assertion to make. Actions speak louder than words. In the age of information, and accessibility, we need to call the lack of awareness and information what it is: not a privilege one is granted, but a choice one is making. When you call a thing what it is, you stand a better chance of doing something constructive about it. In this case, becoming curious enough about experiences other than one's own and then choosing to educate oneself is an available option.

We need to open our eyes, our minds, and our hearts to see what is actually occurring in the world beyond the teeny, tiny space we occupy. It is time to quit referring to a lack of information, knowledge, and awareness as a privilege, and simply call it a lack of information, knowledge, and awareness. It is time to stop claiming White privilege as a way of demonstrating "wokeness," and letting one's actions speak to one's level of awareness. There is no shame in not knowing. The shame is in making excuses for it. We do not have a choice about our country of origin, skin color, or the way we have been socialized. But we do have a choice to educate ourselves about skin-color advantages, ethnicities, races, and cultures other than our own. If you choose not to, you become like the blind sages touching the elephant, seeing only one small aspect of the whole. Yoga, if embraced and practiced comprehensively, can help us open to a broader reality.

PEOPLE OF COLOR

"People of color" is a term that is used to describe groups of people who cannot be identified as White, or who do not identify themselves as being White. In short, the term, simply put, means people who are not White. The custom of classifying people as colors, based on the lightness or darkness of skin tone, is called colorism. Colorism signifies discrimination based on skin color where people are treated differently or assigned status based on the social meanings attached to the color of their skin. Alice Walker was the first to coin the term. As long as cultures attach value to skin color, classifying people as colors, regardless of one's race or ethnicity, whether intentional or not, maintains skin-color hierarchy.

Using actual skin tone as a physical descriptor is different from using it as a classification or label to identify which group you or someone else belongs to, and which group has greater value. Using it as a descriptor can actually be a helpful way of identifying someone, in the same way you might use hair color, eye color, height, or any other physical feature that is helpful in distinguishing one person from the next. Describing physical characteristics as a way of identifying what a person looks like is not discriminatory. Using skin color as a way of classifying someone is. The designation "people of color" is a classification. It in no way helps identify what someone looks like; it simply classifies you as belonging to the group that is not White. Children who have not yet been acculturated to use skin color as a classification can shed some light on the difference between skin color as a descriptor and skin color as a classification.

When he was six years old, a friend's son asked, "Mommy, what color am I?" "What color do you think you are?" "I don't know," he said. So she told him to go get his crayon box so they could find the color that he thought he was. He came back with his box of eight crayons but couldn't find a color that matched his skin tone, so she told him to go get his big box of 64 colors. He brought the big box back and looked and looked and finally found a color he thought matched his skin tone. "What color is this?" His mother told him, "That's apricot." "So, I'm apricot?" "If that's the color you see, yes." "Oh, okay," he said. "Well, what color are you?" he asked. "What color do you think I am?" He began looking for a crayon to match his mother's skin tone and at first pulled out burnt sienna, but that wasn't quite right. Finally, he settled on brown. "I think you're brown. Is that okay?" "If that's the color you see," his mother replied. A few days later she picked him up from school and one of his little classmates got into the back seat of the car and asked, "How come you're White and your Mommy's Black?" Her son replied, "I'm NOT white. I'm apricot. And she's NOT black, she's brown." "Oh," said the little boy. Her son went on to say, "And besides there's only one WHITE person in the whole wide world, and his name is Michael Jackson!"

How do you use the term "people of color"?

DIFFERENCES DIVIDE

An old but culturally sanctioned mindset is that differences divide. In Hindu mythology the Suras and the Asuras were neighbors but neither group was particularly interested in interacting with or getting to know the other. Over time, for a complex set of reasons, the Asuras, which simply means not-Suras, who were at one time revered as gods, came to be described as darker beings, evil spirits, or demons, while the Suras were described as beings of light, as gods. What started out as different and unknown became confused with other, in a negative sense. The story of the Suras and the Asuras is ultimately the story of the demonization of "that which is not like me."

Recognizing difference is as important as discovering similarity. Noting similarities is a good thing—without it human interaction would be impossible. But there must also be consideration of our differences as well. We create an imbalance when we lean toward the belief that we should all think the same, act the same, and look the same. When sameness is emphasized more than difference, we can devolve into conformity. Once that happens, difference becomes a problem and we run the risk of elevating mediocrity and devaluing excellence. We each have an aspect of genius within that deserves to be elevated so that we can fulfill our potential. This requires acknowledging difference as a strength.

Yoga offers the view of the human race as one family. Unlike the Suras and the Asuras, who kept their distance from each other, yoga asks us to join together to get to know, honor, celebrate, and share our different perspectives and lived experiences. This is what the two women who spoke up and then posted the coffee-shop video on social media did. By recognizing and acknowledging each other's racial group differences, they formed an alliance and created an organization dedicated to raising awareness of the harm done to people in racialized cultures, and to highlighting what can be done to advocate for positive change. When we are grounded in our awareness of our connection to one another, each one of us can in our own way:

- acknowledge each other's differences
- affirm each other's differences
- advocate for each other's reality and potential
- appreciate each other's gifts and talents.

INDIVIDUALISM AND MERITOCRACY

Generally speaking, there are two different views of how we perceive the world. One view is that the stress and trauma of one individual is not connected to the stress and trauma of another because we are all independent of one another and leading separate lives. Yoga tells us that we are not separate, that we are interconnected, and that that is the nature of all beings. We are all breathing the same air and we all emanate from the same source. When something affects one of us, it impacts all of us.

There are differences in the way members of dominant and subordinated groups think about individualism and meritocracy. Members of racially dominant groups tend to assume that all they have done and have become is the result of their individual hard work and effort, sometimes with little awareness or acknowledgment of the contributions others have made to their success. For example, I was in an outdoor café having lunch when I overheard a conversation between two gentlemen who were discussing whether or not to pay for their adult children's college education. One gentleman, who was opposed to doing so, explained that his father hadn't paid for his college education and that he had paid for his own. "How'd you do that, through student loans?" the other man asked. "No, I paid out of my own pocket. When I turned 18, my father told me he was no longer obliged legally to support me, so I paid for my own college education. See, when we were kids, my parents sold a lot of property and put the money in trust for my brothers and me, and when we turned 18, we got our trusts, so I paid for college out of my own trust fund."

The belief that I alone have accomplished what I have through my own efforts leaves out all of the preconditions that had to occur to make those accomplishments possible. It reinforces feelings of entitlement, isolation, and disconnection. Without awareness of the contributions others have made to one's success, and without awareness of the barriers to success placed in the way of members of subordinated groups, dominant group members might wonder, "If I can do it, why can't they?"

Most members of subordinated groups tend to believe that their successes and their survival have largely been due to group achievements and sacrifices, not individual effort or talent. This is often expressed as "I stand on the shoulders of all those who came before me to make my successes possible." It is important that we understand and acknowledge these various frames of reference if we are to reach deeper levels of understanding across ethnic, racial, and cultural differences.

THE KLESHAS

Recognizing our ethnic, racial, and cultural identity is important from a psychosocial perspective, but there is a deeper level of identity at our core that is ever present and unchanging, an identity that unites us all. Our individual personal and group identities are social constructs based on cultural norms. These aspects of self are superficial, learned, and changeable. To confuse this surface aspect of self with one's core identity is a mistake. Yoga invites us to awaken to the deepest aspects of self to reveal our true unchanging nature. According to Patanjali's Yoga Sutra 2.3–2.9 (Desikachar 1995), we are unaware of our deepest level of being due to five mental states that block our ability to know our true identity. These mental states are called kleshas, which are, in a manner of speaking, our blind spots. The kleshas are called afflictions, or obstacles to clear perception that keep us from seeing without prejudice, and they are regarded as the main cause of all our pain and suffering. All of us are capable of clear perception, but misapprehension, confused values, rigid attachments, irrational dislikes, and fear stand in the way. All of the obstacles are interrelated, with misapprehension being the source of the other four obstacles.

Avidya—misapprehension—is the state of ignorance that arises when you forget your true nature as a loving, kind, compassionate, empathic, peaceful, generous, and joyful being. All of these qualities are aspects of the core of our being that is constant. Life's many distractions can cover up this core and can cause us to mistake thoughts, feelings, situations, circumstances, and biases—all transient things—for who we are. Forgetting our true nature, which constitutes our commonality, makes it impossible for us to see others as souls on a spiritual journey, and causes us to experience the pain of separation. When you fail to grasp your true self, the stage is set for the other four kleshas—asmita, raga, dvesha, and abhinivesha—to arise.

Asmita—ego—is the false identity you substitute for your true self once you have forgotten that you actually are a spiritual being having a human experience. This constructed self is what we call the ego. It is made up of your self-image and defines itself by your attainments, achievements, status, recognition, and power. It is the personal self. The ego is a necessary construct for human beings to develop as a way of establishing a functional human identity. It is important to know that you are not everyone or everything else, that there are certain human characteristics, gifts, and talents that you alone possess. The ego creates these boundaries. This awareness is experienced as "I'm not you, I'm me; this is not yours, this is mine." We see the beginnings of ego development in children around the age of two. This process continues through childhood and adolescence and into adulthood as we distinguish ourselves personally and professionally. The ego creates boundaries, but it is a constructed identity and was never intended to be confused with who we actually are. It is a stop on the way to remembering our true identity.

The adolescent phase of development ushers in an expanded awareness of self that includes the ability to empathize. As we become acquainted with other individuals who are not like us, we find common ground and begin to realize, "I'm somewhat like you." As we become increasingly mature, we become developmentally ripe for recognizing our spiritual connection to all beings and enter into the awareness that beyond my human experience as a unique individual, "I'm nothing but you." A great deal of suffering is caused when we attach ourselves to our constructed identity of "I'm not you" and cling to the ego's need for approval by continuing to distinguish itself from everyone else. We suffer whenever the ego's needs for aggrandizement are not met. As we mature, the ego is intended to become background, not remain in the foreground. It should never be confused with one's true self.[1]

Raga—attachment—is an outgrowth of ego, and is the act of grasping or clinging to your preferences. We all have preferences. That is not the problem. The problem is rigidly holding onto preferences, as if they are permanent. Doing so keeps you from leaving your comfort zone and stunts your personal and spiritual growth. Treating preferences as entitlements or possessions, as if they are permanent, blinds you to their transient nature. When you are deeply attached to anyone or anything, including your thoughts and beliefs, the fear of change can cause you to feel afraid, tense, and anxious and to cling even more.

Dvesha—aversion—is your avoidance of things you don't like or that are painful. Anything that poses a threat to your false sense of self, your ego, will cause you to reject it, limiting your ability to expand your awareness. Aversions tend to be persistent, even when whatever caused

---

1   The developmental trajectory described is based on Western cultural norms. Cultures that emphasize spiritual development, the connection to all living things, and group identity may follow a different developmental path.

the aversion no longer exists. Traumatic retention is an example of an aversion that prevents present-moment awareness.

Abhinivesha—fear—is our attachment to life itself. When our life ends, we cease to exist. Fear of extinction or being forgotten is an experience shared by nearly all human beings, even those who live in misery. The anticipation of the future, the unknown, and what it might bring causes anxiety. Abhinivesha is essentially clinging to all that you have and all that you have ever known for your security. We know that life itself never ends. But the awareness that our personal life will end causes us to be afraid. Instead of flowing with life and allowing it to live through us and guide us, we cling to it as part of our personal identity.

Cultural kleshas contribute to misapprehension and to our implicit and explicit ethnic and racial biases. The kleshas exist in the body as well as the mind, influencing every thought we have and action we take. Thoughts and actions have consequences, and when influenced by misperceptions that go unnoticed and unchallenged, can result in doing harm. Shining the light of awareness on how we are influenced by the kleshas helps us identify and dissolve their influence. If we reduce the influence of the first klesha, ignorance of our true nature, all the other kleshas dissolve. With consistent practice, over time, fear is replaced with the internal state of love and peacefulness, and this influences our thinking mind and our behavior. But Patanjali warns us not to be confused by temporary states of clarity. The dissolution of the kleshas is an ongoing process that requires vigilance and practices that support self-reflection, in order to keep the kleshas from resurfacing and blinding us to their influence.

Yoga brings us back to our core nature. Restorative Yoga is a practice that helps combat the daily distractions and challenges we face by helping us learn to relax and rest deeply and completely. Because it is practiced in relative stillness and silence, there are fewer distractions than we might experience in a more active practice. It is the practice of being present, connecting to the love and goodness that is within, and finding peace and quiet for your entire being. Restorative Yoga teaches patience and the discipline to remain awake as one becomes increasingly relaxed. The intentional observation of breath, stillness, and silence support a deep level of self-reflective awareness. The contemplative nature of the practice teaches us that beyond the limits of our ego there is a higher state of consciousness that can guide, inform, and protect us.

REFLECTION

20/20 Insight

Dark Girls is a documentary in which various shades of brown-skinned American women of African ancestry describe their experiences of being shunned, bullied, and made to feel inferior because of their dark skin (Berry and Duke 2011). All of the women are beautiful, but they have been made to feel unattractive and unwanted in a culture that has an aversion to certain kinds of differences, regarding them as odd, foreign, threatening, or, even worse, repulsive.

Whether or not we know it, like it, or believe it, deeply embedded culturally accepted stereotypes shape our attitudes toward what is acceptable and what is not, as well as who is acceptable and who is not. Americans have been acculturated to regard certain types of beauty, usually fair skin, straight blond hair, blue eyes, toothpick thin, no curves (except maybe for large breasts), as the standard by which to evaluate women as worthy, beautiful, smart (or not), pleasing, and acceptable. And there are other stereotypes that shape our consciousness and affect our attitudes toward race, ethnicity, religion, body type, gender, political affiliation, gun ownership, physical ability, intellectual prowess, age, and more.

Attitudes operate on two levels—consciously and unconsciously. They reflect our thoughts, influence our words, and manifest in our actions. Our conscious attitudes are made up of what we are aware of and what we choose to believe. Our unconscious attitudes are those knee-jerk reactions and automatic associations that lurk beneath the surface of our awareness. These unconscious attitudes could be entirely incompatible with what we say we believe. We don't deliberately choose our unconscious attitudes; we are obviously not aware of them, and therein lies the problem. Unless you become aware, the unconscious may cause you to say or do things that embarrass you and unintentionally harm other people. We see this all the time in media reports of people being falsely accused of wrongdoing based on their looks alone, or the latest high-profile politician, celebrity, or religious leader who has to publicly apologize for making outrageously offensive remarks about a group of people or about an individual who does not fit their stereotype of acceptability.

There is an ongoing national conversation about how to cultivate attitudes and behaviors that embrace and celebrate all types of difference, and that challenge cultural stereotypes. The yoga community in the United States is an important part of this conversation. The word "yoga" means to connect or to join with. Yoga really is for everybody, not just for those who look a certain way, think a certain way, and act a certain way. We can easily forget this and be lulled into thinking of union as sameness, ignoring the reality and the value of difference.

Some of us have been taught to ignore difference, learning that it does not really matter and should not exist in our minds. But that is delusional. Any observant human being knows that difference does exist and does matter. Ignoring differences might give you a feeling of comfort or security, but it creates disconnection between people and makes intimacy impossible. It also sets you up to be hijacked by unconscious attitudes.

Our attitudes around difference may not always be conscious; if we choose to live a conscious life, we can benefit from checking our attitudes. With awareness, we can rid ourselves of unconscious prejudices and shape our consciousness to be open to, embrace, and celebrate a world that is becoming more varied and expansive every moment. If you are curious and want to learn more about your deep-seated attitudes regarding a variety of differences including race and ethnicity, go to www.implicit.harvard.edu and take the test that reveals your unconscious attitudes about difference. It is a real eye-opener. Remember: 20/20 insight is a precursor to change.

DISCUSSION

Complete the following sentences:

- If I learned about race from my parents, I would believe...
- If I learned about race in school, I would believe...
- If I learned about race from my friends, I would believe...
- If I learned about race from television, I would believe...
- If I learned about skin color from my parents, I would believe...
- If I learned about skin color in school, I would believe...
- If I learned about skin color from my friends, I would believe...
- If I learned about skin color from television, I would believe...

Now ask yourselves these questions:

- Are skin color and race the same?
- What are the foundations of your racial and cultural identity based on?

REFERENCES

Bates, K.G. (2017) "New evidence shows there's still bias against black natural hair." NPR: Code Switch. Accessed on 11/15/2019 at www.npr.org/sections/codeswitch/2017/02/06/512943035/new-evidence-shows-theres-still-bias-against-black-natural-hair.

Bates, K.G. (2018) "The education of Bobby Kennedy—on race." NPR: Code Switch. Accessed on 11/15/2019 at www.npr.org/sections/codeswitch/2018/06/05/616942962/the-education-of-bobby-kennedy-on-race.

Berry, D.C. (Producer, Director) and Duke, B. (Producer, Director) (2011) *Dark Girls*. United States: Duke Media/Urban Winter Entertainment.

Bynum, E.B. (2012) *Dark Light Consciousness: Melanin, Serpent Power, and the Luminous Matrix of Reality*. Rochester, VT: Inner Traditions International.

Desikachar, T.K.V. (1995) *The Heart of Yoga: Developing a Personal Practice*. Rochester, VT: Inner Traditions International.

Liu, W.M., Liu, R.Z., Garrison, Y.L., Kim, J.Y.C., *et al.* (2019) "Racial trauma, microaggressions, and becoming racially innocuous: The role of acculturation and white supremacist ideology." *American Psychologist 74*, 1, 143–155.

Martin, A. (2017) "The hatred of black hair goes beyond ignorance." *Time*, August 23, 2017. Accessed on 11/15/2019 at https://time.com/4909898/black-hair-discrimination-ignorance.

Merriam-Webster (2019) "Classical." Accessed on 11/15/2019 at www.merriam-webster.com/dictionary/classical.

Solomon, A. (2013) "Depression, the Secret We Share." TEDxMet. Accessed on 11/15/2019 at www.ted.com/talks/andrew_solomon_depression_the_secret_we_share?language=en.

West, R.T. (2018) "Lost Shadow." Ronald Thomas West, blog post, April 6, 2018. Accessed on 11/15/2019 at https://ronaldthomaswest.com/2018/04/06/lost-shadow.

Willon, P. and Díaz, A. (2019) "California becomes first state to ban discrimination based on one's natural hair." *Los Angeles Times*, July 3, 2019. Accessed on 11/15/2019 at www.latimes.com/local/lanow/la-pol-ca-natural-hair-discrimination-bill-20190703-story.html.

Chapter 6

COMMUNITIES OF CARE

WHEN YOU live in a culture that emphasizes autonomy and independence over interdependence, you can lose sight of the fact that you are wired to live in connection with others. Currently, there is what researchers are calling a loneliness epidemic in the United States. But the U.S. is not alone. Sweden, the United Kingdom, Japan, Italy, Canada, Russia, South Africa, Kenya, and Brazil are also listed in the top ten loneliest countries in the world (Brannan 2019). People complain of feeling left out, of not having companionship, and that no one knows them well. This kind of social isolation poses a risk to emotional and physical health and well-being. The problem of loneliness, as it turns out, is not age-related and is affecting both young and old alike. We are not meant to live in isolation. We are social beings, created to live in loving connection with one another. We are mothers, fathers, wives, husbands, sisters, brothers, daughters, sons, friends, neighbors, and co-workers. Creating caring community is one way to mitigate the harm done by social disconnection and isolation from other people.

Community is not a location, an organization, or a place where people gather. Community is a sense of connection and relationship among people with shared needs, interests, and common goals, designed to meet the common needs of community members. Members of a community have a sense of trust and belonging and feel safe in the presence of one another. They care for each other and feel empowered to contribute to the health and well-being of one another by creating environments that are loving, welcoming, supportive, and physically and emotionally safe. Community is a heartfelt experience. It is not about diversity, inclusion, or exclusion. It is not about agreement or conformity. It is not about dogma or political ideology. It is about loving relationship, connection, collaboration, openness, and warmth, and doing the work that supports all of this.

"Kula" is a Sanskrit term that means community of the heart. It represents a community of yogis who come together with intention and a shared purpose. Intentional yoga communities formed to address and heal the wounds of ethnic and racial distress are communities of love that focus on self-care for the benefit of the entire community, not just for those who have had direct experiences of racial wounding. These are communities that recognize that the health and well-being of those who experience ongoing, cumulative, and recurrent race-based stress and trauma is the responsibility of all. These are communities that understand that we owe our selfhood to each other and that no man, woman, or child stands alone. These communities are not necessarily, but can be, multiracial, multicultural, multiethnic, and global as well, and they are voluntary.

There is an African proverb that says one finger cannot pick up a grain. It means that some things, no matter how simple they might appear, require the cooperation and help of others to accomplish a goal. And so it is with communities of care. Individuals who stand alone are never as effective as those who share and honor the consciousness of the Ubuntu philosophy "I am because we are." As it relates to ethnic and race-based stress and trauma, these are yoga communities that support those who are targets of ethnic and racial discrimination, violence and injustice, and the allies who advocate for them. There are also communities that support examining one's own ethnic and racial bias to unlearn old ways of thinking and behaving. These are communities that recognize that both the individuals who are the targets of racial wounding and those who perpetuate it need help. The support is mutual and reciprocal. Two such communities come to mind. At a yoga training designed to address the issues of racial trauma, in a community that experienced the devastating death of one of its young members to gun violence at the hands of law enforcement, the host mentioned that the allies in their yoga kula were providing childcare for parents who wanted to attend the training. Another example is of an innovative yoga therapist and studio owner who regards herself as a racial and social justice activist. Rather than focusing on diversity and inclusion initiatives, she intuited the need for her community of practitioners to work with their internalized racial biases, and she began to offer yoga classes and workshops on the theme of racial bias awareness to those who were ready and interested in this process.

Caring communities are a reflection of the collective consciousness that binds them together. When you feel a sense of love, belonging, and solidarity based on the norms, habits, and customs that support the awareness that we are human first, and that I am because we are, you are able to form communities that are not hierarchical but that reflect a consciousness of connection and collaboration. There are individual differences in caring communities and there are disagreements too. But there is a willingness to communicate with each other, to honor one another's uniqueness, context, life experience, and cultural, racial, and ethnic identities, and to work toward understanding various perspectives whenever there is disagreement. Individuals within the community take more than themselves into consideration. They take into consideration what benefits or harms the whole before putting their own needs and interests first. There is acknowledgment and awareness of we, not just me. The consciousness of "I am because we are" understands that the relationships within the community are equal to or greater than whatever issue comes up or whatever task needs to be done. Connection comes first. Self-care is understood as action that is done in service of supporting a healthy, caring community. It is not an act of selfishness or of self-indulgence. Self-care is engaged in, so that members of the community can take good care of each other. Feeling taken care of is an important aspect of healing from ethnic and race-based stress and trauma. Caring for self, caring for others, and being taken care of are reciprocal acts. Reciprocity and mutuality, giving and receiving, are energies that, when balanced within us individually, permeate consciousness and are expressed as shared responsibility for the well-being of all.

Race-based stress and trauma are real, and result in experiences of emotional harm caused by various forms of social disconnection and exclusion. What makes racial stress and trauma unique is the context in which it occurs. There is an external context and an internal context, an actual event and an emotional experience. Our focus is on the internal experiences associated with race-related events and how connection, Restorative Yoga, and sharing our stories with one another can contribute to easing the suffering of racial wounding and support repair, restoration, resilience, recovery, and mental clarity. Every human being is an expression of one's own inner experience. When our inner experience is in alignment and in harmony with our core self, this is mirrored in our consciousness and is reflected in our body, emotions, mind, relationships, and all that we say or do. It brings us into harmony with the principle of Ubuntu which becomes a lived experience, not just words on a page. This does not just happen. It must be conscious and intentional. Yoga provides the foundation for creating and living in conscious and intentionally caring community.

THE FOUNDATION OF CARING COMMUNITY

Patanjali's Yoga Sutra identifies an eightfold path to living life consciously with meaning, depth, and purpose. Each path directs attention toward one's physical, mental, emotional, and spiritual health and well-being, and includes ten guidelines for ethical conduct and self-regulation called yamas and niyamas. Yamas and niyamas are not commandments but are aspects of our true nature when we are centered in the core of our being. Patanjali tells us that yamas and niyamas are qualities of goodness that we all share. The illusion of separateness is what causes us to behave in ways that are contrary to our true nature. As our yoga practice deepens, the illusion of separateness dissolves and we realize that at the core level of being there is no "other," no difference between you and me. What happens to one happens to all.

In ancient times, when the contemplative practices of yoga were primary, it was expected that one attain a certain level of mastery over the yamas and niyamas before engaging in the six pathways that followed; yamas and niyamas, asana, pranayama, and the three pathways toward meditation. Current yoga practices in the Western Hemisphere do not always emphasize the yamas, niyamas, and contemplative practices, and instead have become more focused on the physical practices of yoga. In spite of the shift in focus, T.K.V. Desikachar tells us that regardless of an individual's reasons for practicing yoga or for a preferred entry point into the practice, whether it be asana, pranayama, or meditation, as one engages in a consistent practice and progresses, each of the eightfold paths of yoga develops simultaneously (Desikachar 1995). This makes the entry point or the order of practice less important than the actual practice itself. He reminds us that in order to sustain living by the yamas and niyamas, we must embody them and experience them as part of us, not regard them as merely aspirational ideals or commandments to follow.

As one embraces yoga as a lifestyle, more than just a physical exercise or a relaxation technique, the ten ethical observances can be the foundation of conscious communities of care and connection. What if in addition to using our energy to figure out how to create more diversity and inclusion within yoga communities, we focused on creating caring communities based on the ten ethical principles of Pantanjali's Yoga Sutra, by making a commitment to actually be the principles? Not only can the five yamas serve as guides for individual behavior in relationship to self, others, and the environment, they can also serve as guides that can be used to envision and lay the groundwork for creating the kind of yoga community you would like to be a part of. The five niyamas can serve as guides that support one's internal practices of self-care and spiritual development that are essential to conscious, caring, connected, and collaborative community.

Living the yamas and niyamas supports open-heartedness, compassion, generosity, and serenity, in keeping with what the yogis tell us are aspects of our true nature. They apply to one's individual thoughts, words, and behavior, and apply to living in community. They are expressed in ways that are unique to each individual member and serve as guides for using your energy to develop character, build community, live in harmony with each other, and evolve spiritually.

YAMAS

Our attitude and how we relate to others and the external world is called yama. The way we behave toward others and our environment reflects our perceptions, shaped by our personality, our life experiences, and cultural conditioning as well as our racial and ethnic identity, among many other influences. Unexamined, these external influences can create obstacles to clear perception, causing us to make errors in judgment as to who we actually are and in how we relate to others. As we practice asana, pranayama, and meditation, we become more observant of our attitudes and behaviors toward others and our environment. We are then better able to correct the flaws in our perceptions and to adopt and sustain the attitudes that reflect our true nature from the depth of our being.

AHIMSA—NON-HARMING

Sutra 2.35 is the first of the disciplines described in Patanjali's Yoga Sutra and is the cornerstone of the other nine observances. It means leading a life that does not harm other living beings, including one's self. This is not limited to physical harm, but includes harmful thoughts, attitudes, words, and actions as well. Starting with self is important because we cannot treat others any better than we treat ourselves. This means that in order to develop loving relationships with others, self-love must become part of our consciousness and our practice. It means we must be committed to doing no harm to ourselves by refraining from thinking negatively of ourselves, including calling ourselves names in frustration or anger. It means letting go of shame, blame, and criticism of ourselves, and not engaging in any behavior that is in any way harmful to our physical body, emotional body, mental body, or spiritual body. It means treating ourselves with respect, kindness, and compassion, and making peace with ourselves in order to make peace with others and with the world at large.

Causing harm to one's self or others is a form of withholding love and is usually based on fear. Whenever you find yourself fearful, before acting ask yourself, "What is the most loving thing I can do for myself, my loved one, or the person standing in front of me in this moment?" Remember love is a choice we make and an action we take, not an emotion we feel. Emotion is fleeting. Feelings cannot be relied on when it comes to being loving, because feelings can change in an instant. When we decide to be loving to self or to others, we are not relying on emotion, likes, or dislikes. We are engaged in a disciplined practice of non-harming. Love takes intention and effort. It does not just happen. We do not have to feel loving to be loving but we do have to be intentional. Do not be afraid to love too much for fear of being hurt or for fear of loss. Loving others and loving self are reciprocal acts. When you learn to love yourself for who you are, not for who someone else needs you to be, you can love others the same way. This is how we do no harm.

SATYA—TRUTHFULNESS

Sutra 2.36, satya, is the second of the ten yamas and niyamas. It is the ability to be honest with one's self and with others, without being brutal. It has been said that brutal honesty is more brutal than honest. Some people pride themselves on being brutally honest, while others avoid being honest for fear of being hurtful. Neither extreme is optimal. There is a middle way. Being honest requires a measure of discernment if it is to be expressed skillfully. A beloved client gave me a plaque that hangs on my wall as I enter my meditation room and serves as an important reminder of the principle of satya. It is attributed to Sai Baba and cautions that before you speak, ask yourself, "Is it true? Is it kind? Is it necessary? Does it improve upon the silence?" If you follow this guidance, you will speak the truth to others with integrity and with kindness.

Being truthful with one's self starts by being open to the truth of your own being. What that means is being willing to know who you are and to be who you are. We have all been gifted with unique talents and are duty-bound to use our gifts to create meaningful, purposeful lives. To ignore, reject, or misuse your innate abilities is a violation of the truth. In a passage from the ancient text, the *Bhagavad Gita*, on the eve of an epic battle, in a conversation between Arjuna, a great but reluctant warrior, and Krishna, the lord disguised as Arjuna's charioteer, Krishna instructs Arjuna that "It is better to strive in one's own dharma than to succeed in someone else's" (Easwaran 2000, p.21). Another way of saying this is: be true to your calling. You cannot be someone else better than you can be yourself. If you are unsure of what your gifts and talents are, or what your calling is, spend some time paying attention to what comes naturally to you. What interests you most? This is where your strengths and abilities lie. Then spend time reflecting on how to best use your talent for the good of others. It may not seem like it, but as you honor your own truth, you will find the courage and the wisdom to be truthful with others without being cruel. Rather than competing with one another, in conscious caring communities, members support one another in discovering and utilizing their unique gifts and talents for the benefit of all.

ASTEYA—NON-STEALING

Sutra 3.7, asteya, is the third of the yamas and niyamas. It is an important aspect of self-love and of a loving community. Asteya means honoring boundaries and not coveting, envying, or taking what does not belong to you. Taking what does not belong to you manifests in many different ways. It can range from something as obvious as robbing a bank or shoplifting, to something subtler such as taking credit for someone else's idea, stealing someone's joy, taking up more space than you need, taking advantage of someone's time, or wasting someone's money.

I learned an important lesson about taking what did not belong to me and the value of caring community early on as a child. One day, when I was about ten years old, I found a five-dollar bill in our neighbor's driveway. I picked it up, put it in my pocket, and went to the corner store. I bought myself some candy, two comic books, and had change to spare for another spending spree. When I arrived home with my purchases, my mother asked me where I had gotten the money to buy them. When I told her I found the money in the neighbor's driveway, she explained to me that the five-dollar bill was not mine but was probably our neighbor's, and told me I made a mistake by not asking our neighbor if she had lost the money before I decided to take it and spend it. She asked me what I thought we should do. We agreed we should go back to the store together, explain what happened, see if I could return the items, and get the money back. Then we should go next door to ask our neighbor if she had lost the five dollars. This is exactly what we did. And guess what? The neighbor was so grateful, as a reward, she gave me the five dollars to keep. That was an incredibly important lesson in kindness, generosity, the value of truthfulness, and not taking something that did not belong to me. When we practice asteya, the real reward is the experience of the benevolence and abundance of the universe.

Another form of taking is robbing someone of their cultural, racial, or ethnic identity. We do harm when we expect others to be like us and shame, ridicule, or bully them for not conforming to our expectations. The same is true when we appropriate culture. We show disrespect and do harm when we do not bother to cultivate knowledge, skills, and competence in dealing with a culture other than our own, or take what is not ours without giving credit to or showing appreciation and respect for the culture we are emulating or taking from.

Envy is another form of taking what is not yours. I want what you have, or I want to be who you are. We erroneously think that having what we don't have will alleviate our suffering, not realizing that it is focusing on what we do not have, not the absence of the thing, that causes our suffering. As long as you compare yourself with others as being better or worse off than you are, you will suffer, and you will deprive yourself of the peacefulness and contentment that is your birthright. Wanting to be who you are and wanting what you have are important manifestations of asteya.

BRAHMACHARYA—MODERATION

Sutra 2.38, brahmacharya, is the fourth of the yamas and niyamas. It is about merging our sensual nature with the divine to create balance. In a material world we can become so focused on the physical aspects of existence that we neglect or ignore our spiritual nature. We are sensate beings and without a measure of moderation can become addicted to sensation. If we are not being stimulated or feeling something strongly, we may be inclined to ramp up the intensity in our quest to feel more. One of our strongest sensual urges is our sexual urge. Brahmacharya is the decision to exercise self-control when it comes to indulging our sensual, including our sexual, urges. The intention is not to deny our physical nature or to deprive ourselves of pleasure, but instead to channel our sensual energy to be used in service of cultivating and deepening the development of our spiritual nature. When we honor and live by the five yamas—ahimsa/non-harming, satya/truthfulness, asteya/non-stealing, brahmacharya/moderation, and the fifth yama, aparigraha/non-attachment—we are doing just that.

A dear friend and fellow yogini shares a story that illuminates the practice of exercising this ethical restraint. A sage places a beautiful bejeweled urn in front of his students and asks them to look at it. After a time, he asks who would like to have the urn. Then he asks what they would be willing to do to possess the urn. Finally, he points out that when we move from just seeing the urn, to wanting the urn, to taking action to possess the urn, we are using energy in ways that can distract us from nourishing our spiritual nature. He ends the lesson by asking, "Can you just see and appreciate the urn?" When you can just see an object, and appreciate the object without having to possess it, you are exercising restraint.

Brahmacharya is the utilization of your energy to see beyond the physical and the sensual, and to see the divinity in all. The practice of brahmacharya invites you to nurture your own and one another's spiritual growth. When we overindulge in sensual pleasures, we are externally focused and distract ourselves from doing the inner work of spiritual development. The consequence of spiritual neglect appears as symptoms of depression, addictions, violence, obsessions, feelings of emptiness, and loss of meaning. When we try to make ourselves feel better by eradicating these symptoms or by indulging in material excess, we do more harm than good. We might try to ease our sense of lack with food, possessions, sex, drugs, alcohol, work, exercise, even asana and meditation. When none of these remedies work, we erroneously think more will be better. Erring on the side of indulging our physical desires, we become imbalanced. No amount of material excess can fill a spiritual need. We fail to nurture our spiritual nature by trying to relieve our suffering through physical indulgences. By withdrawing your attention from your senses, and shifting to an internal focus, you can use your energy to nurture your soul and achieve a balance between your physical and spiritual nature.

In caring community, each of us has the freedom to find and then practice what nourishes one's soul. Brahmacharya doesn't ask us to ignore or deny the physical aspects of our being; rather, it invites us to regard our body, mind, and soul as aspects of the divine and to behave accordingly. One size never fits all. For some it might be a religious practice, for others it might be a meditation practice, and still others might find music, dance, writing, the visual or performing arts, communing in nature, or intimate relationships to be nourishment for the soul.

One way to nourish the soul is to notice and honor the sacred in the everydayness of life; those ordinary things you don't normally pay attention to because they are routine, such as home, family, friendships, community, what you eat, the clothes you wear—in other words, your mundane daily activities. Paying attention to life's small details through the lens of the sacred gives depth and meaning to our lives in ways that excess and indulgence never can. In her novel *The Color Purple*, Alice Walker's description of God being "pissed off" "when you pass by the color purple in a field without noticing it" (Walker 1983, p.191) is a reminder to notice the sacred in the ordinary. To merge our consciousness with the divine is to notice the color purple, to notice the sunset, to notice the clouds in the sky and the mud puddle in the dirt left by rainfall, and then to notice the delight that fills you just because you noticed. As you do this, you begin to realize that the divine resides in all beings, and that everything is reciprocal. You begin to realize that it is not just pleasing the divine that matters. It is the awareness that the divine wants to please us too. It is the merging of our energies with the divine that allows us to experience the sacred in ourselves and in all of life. When we abuse the sacred by ignoring it or by overindulgence, we violate brahmacharya. So brahmacharya means merging our energies with the divine to discover the sacredness in all of life, even in the ordinary. When this happens, it changes our relationship to everyone and everything. The paradox is that by noticing the sacred in the ordinary, we experience the extraordinary.

APARIGRAHA—NON-ATTACHMENT

Sutra 2.39, aparigraha, is the fifth of the yamas and niyamas. It has to do with accepting change. Change is inevitable. No matter how much we wish that things would remain the same, and no matter how hard we try to ensure that they do, that is not the way life works. Summer becomes fall, fall becomes winter, winter becomes spring, day becomes night, and young becomes old. That is the way of nature. Our resistance to change prevents us from growing and living life in a dynamic and enjoyable way.

Aparigraha is the practice of surrendering to the inevitability of change. Holding onto the way we want life to be instead of accepting life on its own terms, moment to moment, means letting go of what was, and accepting what is occurring in the moment. It doesn't mean we won't be disappointed, or sad, angry, resistant, or even afraid sometimes when change is required. Those feelings are normal and natural. But it means releasing what was and looking to the future with excitement and the anticipation of possibilities and opportunities for growth as well.

Even though growth can be uncomfortable and sometimes even downright painful, the pain of transition is not nearly as painful as holding onto what needs to be let go. It is normal and natural to contract around a painful loss, for example. But remaining in a contracted state goes against the natural rhythm of change. When you breathe in, you naturally breathe out. The simple act of paying attention to breath is a powerful lesson in the wisdom and necessity of letting go. You can also feel this in your body when you stretch, relax, and then let go. It actually feels good. Think about some of the things you cling to: material objects, moments, status, power, control, youth, grudges, resentments, beliefs, opinions, relationships, to name a few. All of these can be let go.

As racial and ethnic demographics in various nations and communities around the world change, are you willing to make the shifts necessary to embrace multiracial, multiethnic multiculturalism as a reality? Are you willing to make the necessary adjustments to accommodate the changes this reality brings? What do you have to let go of to do so? When we accept the inevitability of change, we learn to trust the process of life and begin to discover that no matter how difficult the transition is that life asks us to make, after all is said and done, life really is on our side. Caring community can help us understand this.

NIYAMAS

While yamas are concerned with our relationship to the world, niyamas are concerned with our inner observances and are evidence of living one's best life. Niyamas are manifestations of living up to the highest expressions of one's being.

SAUCHA—PURITY

Sutra 2.40, saucha, is the sixth of the yamas and niyamas. It is purification of our mind, body, and environment. The ancient yogis understood that in order to maximize our ability to be free of disease, obtain mental clarity, gain wisdom, and experience inner freedom, we need to optimize behaviors that support this. They understood that what we take into our body and mind, the state of our living conditions, and the quality of our relationships all have an impact on our physical, emotional, and mental health. The practice of saucha is the practice of cleanliness that supports overall health and well-being. This means making the effort to eat clean food, uncontaminated by pesticides and unnatural chemicals, drinking clean water, and reading books and enjoying various forms of entertainment that inspire. It means living in an orderly, clean, uncluttered environment, and choosing relationships that are non-toxic as well.

Saucha might reveal itself in your life in many ways. You might be purifying your relationships—maybe letting go of some toxic people in your life to make room for something new. You might be purifying your body by ridding it of toxic substances and releasing toxic behaviors such as overindulgence in unhealthy foods and beverages. You might be maintaining a regimen of physical fitness that helps purify and release toxic substances from your body. You might be purifying your mind of thoughts of hatred, jealousy, hostility, negativity, revenge. You might be purifying your environment by letting go of items that no longer serve or have a place in your life, that are taking up space and making your environment look cluttered. You might be advocating for environmental policies that support health and well-being. When we engage in the process of cleansing with loving kindness, patience, and awareness, we reduce our suffering. How does saucha reveal itself in your life?

Santosha—Contentment

Sutra 2.41, santosha, is the seventh of the yamas and niyamas. It is the observance that seems to meet with the most resistance in the Western Hemisphere. Many people confuse contentment with complacency, but this could not be further from the truth. Simply put, contentment is wanting what you have. In a consumer culture, where having what you want is the focus, this one is hard to fathom and harder to master. Think about it this way. Getting what you want does not matter as long as you keep striving to get what you do not have. No matter how much you have, there will always be more of what you do not have than what you do have, so striving for more becomes a vicious cycle. Once you stop focusing on what you don't have, and start appreciating what you already have, you feel content, satisfied, fulfilled, and peaceful. Does that mean you will never have more? No. It just means that when you're content, you stop asking for what you don't have and start wanting what you do have. Practices of gratitude and appreciation lead to contentment. The more content you are with what you have, the more joyful and happy you become. When we are content, we are free from the suffering that comes from a sense of lack, and we become more aware of the abundance that surrounds us. We begin to feel full in our being, so we no longer have to rely on externals for a sense of completeness. This is hardly complacency.

Contentment reveals itself in your life in many ways. It can be the fulfillment that comes from taking a walk in nature, resting in the sun, petting your dog or cat, or hugging someone you love. It might come from eating a good meal without feeling full and bloated, or being in community with others who are learning something about themselves. One of the keys to contentment is living in the moment, not being focused on the past or the future, or what else you could or should be doing, or who else you could or should be with. It means not looking outside yourself for happiness or fulfillment. It means doing what you love and loving what you do. It means loving the one you're with—you—whether or not you are with the one you love. How does santosha reveal itself in your life?

Tapas—Inner Heat

Sutra 2.42, tapas, is the eighth of the yamas and niyamas. In Sanskrit, tapas means heat. It is the determination and passion to create a life built on the principles of the eight-limbed path of yoga, and the willingness to go through whatever discomfort it takes to do so. Tapas is discipline. It asks us to devote ourselves to living the yamas and niyamas, to asana practice, pranayama practices, and meditation practices, whether we want to or not. It asks us to be loving, whether or not we feel loving, to be truthful, whether or not we want to be, and then to find a way to tell the truth skillfully. It asks us to purify our thoughts and our relationships, to stand in the fire of our own impatience when we think we cannot wait one moment longer. Tapas is what helps us put relationships ahead of self. It helps us keep our mouths shut when we want to prove our point and be right at the expense of someone else or of the relationship. Tapas is not for the weak-hearted. It is hard!

Tapas reminds us of our soul's yearning to be free of the attachments that imprison us, our stuff, including attitudes, beliefs, material possessions, and habits. It fuels and directs our spiritual energy. It is the part of you that just keeps you showing up on your yoga mat, on your meditation cushion, in your truth, in your compassion, in your wisdom, because you've made a commitment to remain true to your heart's deepest desire to do so, not because you are being coerced but because you cannot help it. With laser-like intensity, tapas invites us to pay attention. When we are in conflict because our thinking mind or our bodily urges want something contrary to our commitment to living our yoga, tapas is the internal fire that helps us stay on the path. Tapas helps build and fortify our willpower and directs our energy inward. It keeps us from being distracted away from being true to the core of our being. Tapas reveals itself in your life as a willingness to do the needful spiritual practices, to remain faithful to your core, not because you necessarily want to, but because you must.

An example of tapas in action is the commitment of the yoga studio owner, mentioned earlier in this chapter, to remain steadfast in her desire to combine racial and social justice activism with yoga practices and to offer them in her studio. In her courageous commitment to do so, she naively assumed that others would enthusiastically embrace her vision. She was stunned and traumatized by the hateful responses she initially received for her efforts in the form of internet trolling, negative media coverage, and even death threats. Rather than retreating into oblivion, or seeking revenge, she remains dedicated to transforming the consciousness of those members of the community who are interested in learning to examine their racial and ethnic bias, through the practice of yoga. She still faces criticism, but tapas helps her stand in the heat of all of this without being intimidated or burning out. Being an advocate requires tapas! How does tapas reveal itself in your life?

SVADHYAYA—SELF-STUDY

Sutra 2.43, svadhyaya, is the ninth of the yamas and niyamas. According to the yogis, knowing one's true self is the path to liberation. At some point on the yogic path we begin to ask, "Who am I?" This question tends to arise spontaneously, often during periods of transition. One of the more memorable times this question arose for me was about six months before I closed my psychotherapy practice. I had been in the practice for 40 years and was contemplating closing it. I could tell the time was drawing near, but I had not yet decided. I was struggling because after 40 years as a practicing psychologist I wanted to be certain I was ready. It had become my habit to check in with myself daily in my meditation for internal guidance to make sure that I was. In one meditation a question popped into my mind that I was unable to ignore: "Who will I be if I'm not Dr. Gail Parker?" It literally took my breath away. All I could do was sit still and just be with it. Until that moment, I had not realized the extent to which my identity was tied up in my professional role and title. It was my yoga practice that offered me a pathway into my interior life, taking me into a deeper exploration of this question in a way that psychology never could. Psychology, through analysis, can help us understand why we are triggered, what past experiences influence our current behavior, and why we think the way we do, but svadhyaya invites us to go deeper into the inquiry to know who we truly are at our core, beyond the mind's explanations. It takes us beyond studying about the personal self and invites us to uncover the true self and to answer the question "Who am I?" from the depth of our being.

Svadhyaya involves the use of mantra, chanting, the study of ancient texts, inspirational wisdom, contemplation, self-reflection, introspection, and meditation to answer the question "Who am I?" It is best described as self-reflective awareness. This takes time and commitment and a willingness to go deep. As I remained in meditation, I remembered the greeting of the women at the water pump in Cameroon who said, "I am alive and well and in my skin. My soul is in my body." They did not say,

"I am my skin, I am my body." They said, "I am my soul." When all of our attachments and superficial identities fall away, we can answer with sincerity, "I am the one who notices. I am the witnessing awareness of my being. I am that which never changes. I am my soul." When you become established in the seat of self, you realize that you are not your body, emotions, or thoughts. Yes, you have all three, but it is not who you are. You are not your titles, accomplishments, successes, or failures. You are not free from suffering; you are the one who observes your suffering, the one who notices the injustices in the world, the one who faces challenges and who sits compassionately with others in their pain and suffering. You are the consciousness that is experiencing all of this. When this becomes your identity, you know who you are. Svadhyaya is the pathway. How does svadhyaya reveal itself in your life?

ISHVARA PRANIDHANA—SURRENDER TO YOUR HIGHER POWER

Sutra 2.44, Ishvara Pranidhana, is the tenth of the yamas and niyamas. It invites us to surrender to love and to the divinity in ourselves and in all beings. It teaches that through the process of surrender, beyond the limits of our ego, there is a higher state of consciousness that guides, informs, and protect us. It invites us to let go of our attachment to the mind as our sole authority and to open to spirit as our guide. Each of the yamas and niyamas has prepared us to become devoted to experiencing ourselves and all beings as an aspect of the divine. It does not mean giving up our personal identity; rather, it means devoting ourselves to stepping into love as our true identity.

When my son was about three years old, one day, in all of his three-year-old wisdom, he declared with such sweetness, "I love you, Mommy. You are love." It was the first time it occurred to me that I am love. It is a contemplation that I cherish and practice to this day. As I contemplated the question, who would I be if I'm not Dr. Gail Parker, I remembered, I am love. Established in the identity of "I am love," this identity becomes the guiding principle of one's life.

Embodying the yamas and niyamas is different from espousing them as virtuous. They are virtues, of course, but our yoga practice helps us become the embodiment of these virtues. This takes intention, time, and commitment. Envision a community of people dedicated to the awareness of themselves and each other as the embodiment of love. What does it look like? What does it feel like? How does Ishvara Pranidhana reveal itself in your life?

CREATING CARING COMMUNITY

I recently had a conversation with a young yogini who said she has yet to find a yoga community that offers what she is looking for. She said, "I guess I'll just keep looking." She was not talking about asana; she was talking about connection, a community of care. But she was looking outside of herself for the community she longed for, not within. One of my sheroes, visionary, author, and Nobel laureate, Toni Morrison, said she began to write because no one had written the books she wanted to read, so she engaged her imagination to create. Imagination is an internal process. It is not a function of the thinking analytical mind. The thinking mind is a storehouse of information and in our attempts to problem-solve and to increase our knowledge, our tendency is to gather more information. Gathering information has its place, but its focus is external and therefore limited. In Western cultures, we tend to give the thinking mind priority, but in a creative process the thinking mind does not come first—imagination does. Imagination is not a function of the thinking mind. It is a function of a deeper, interior, intuitive level of knowing. To create, we must open to grace and surrender to the realm of the unseen, the unknown, and allow it to reveal itself to us. This is where imagination resides. Become internally focused before you become externally directed. Contemplative practices and Restorative Yoga, which is a contemplative practice, support an internal focus. If you have not yet found the yoga community to which you would like to belong, stop looking to other people to create it for you. First, look within. What kind of community would you create? What if through your yoga practice you began to embody and become your vision? What if you clarified the role you want to play? With the yamas and niyamas as guides, yoga serves us by inviting transformation rather than by providing information. Living the yamas and niyamas and a Restorative Yoga practice are nurturing ways to embrace an idea and to create an internal environment that allows your vision of caring community to take root, blossom, and grow.

REFLECTION

Make a Way Out of No Way

There is a popular urban legend that circulates about Itzhak Perlman, one of the greatest and most famous violinists of our time. He contracted polio as a child, requiring him to wear leg braces and to walk with crutches. Now, at each concert performance, he makes a slow entrance on his crutches onto the stage, sits down, unclasps the braces on his legs, and prepares to play. As the story goes, one evening in a performance at New York's Lincoln Center, he entered the stage in his usual way and began performing a challenging concerto. Near the middle of the performance, one of the strings on his violin broke. Everyone in the audience could hear the loud snap. For any other violinist, this would not have been a problem—embarrassing maybe, but not a problem. He would have simply gotten up, gone to the side of the stage, and attached a new string or gotten another violin. The audience sat in silence waiting to see what Perlman would do. Would he have to put his braces back on and painstakingly make his way across the stage to find another violin?

They watched in wonder as he paused, closed his eyes, and remained still. Then he signaled for the conductor to begin again. Perlman picked up where he had left off and began passionately playing the piece in its entirety with only three strings. It was obvious watching him that he was creating, modulating, and reconfiguring the piece in his head to accommodate the absent string. At the end of the performance, there was an awed silence. Then the audience went wild, jumping to their feet in deafening applause. Perlman raised his bow to quiet the crowd. When the audience settled down, he spoke in a reverent tone. "You know," he said, "sometimes it is the artist's task to find out how much music you can still make with what you have left."

Grandmothers used to call that making do with what you have, or making a way out of no way. In yoga, making do with what you have, or finding a way out of no way, is one of ten ethical principles practiced to cultivate inner harmony and strength. It is called the practice of santosha, or contentment. To the yogi, practicing contentment is a wise way of making peace with your family, your community, and yourself. It is a pathway to joy and a way of becoming satisfied within the container of your own experience. It involves the practice of appreciating and wanting what you have instead of focusing your attention on having what you want.

Contentment should not be confused with complacency, which is a state of stagnation, or no growth. Rather, contentment is a sign that we are at peace with our circumstances and ourselves. Being content does not mean that we have to settle for what we do not want, whether it is a toxic relationship, unbearable living conditions, or inhumane treatment. Contentment starts with accepting reality as it is, not as we want it to be. Accepting reality can lead us to make the necessary changes that result in an overall sense of well-being.

Paradoxically, accepting reality as it is can help us develop a greater capacity for hopefulness. It opens us to the possibility of a better situation than the one we may find ourselves in. The Perlman parable teaches us that by accepting reality as it is, instead of longing for something different, we can learn to make something beautiful with what we have left.

Contentment is not the same as happiness. We all face difficult times in our lives. But it is possible to find contentment even in painful circumstances through acceptance of the situation. In the case of a devastating illness, loss, or other unwelcome circumstance, we may go through various stages of emotional turmoil such as denial, anger, and depression before we reach acceptance. But it is possible to find contentment and inner peace, even then.

No matter what your situation, there is always the possibility of living life more fully. Contentment is the ability to appreciate how much you have, rather than how much you want. As we cultivate this attitude within ourselves, we become more stable in our ability to remain joyful, even when things don't go as we planned or as we hoped they would. When we find a way to make do with what we have, we have opened the door to making a way out of no way, to finding peace and contentment within ourselves, and to becoming joyful beyond measure.

DISCUSSION

- What does your ideal caring yoga space, community, or organization look like?

- Who would be represented?
- Why is this important to you?
- What is one thing you are willing to do to create the kind of space, community, or organization you would like to see?
- What is the outcome you are trying to create?
- What influence do you have to affect the outcome you are trying to create?

REFERENCES

Brannan, A. (2019) "The top ten loneliest countries in the world." Immigroup: Immigration News. Accessed on 11/18/2019 at www.immigroup.com/news/top-10-loneliest-countries-world.

Desikachar, T.K.V. (1995) *The Heart of Yoga: Developing a Personal Practice.* Rochester, VT: Inner Traditions International.

Easwaran, E. (2000) *The Bhagavad Gita.* New York, NY: Vintage Books.

Walker, A. (1983) *The Color Purple.* Orlando, FL: Harcourt Brace Jovanovich.

Chapter 7

SPIRITUAL ACTIVISM— YOGA FROM THE INSIDE OUT

YOGA IS a path to self-discovery that leads you to come into direct contact with your spiritual nature. That was its original intended purpose. The quest of the Rishis during the pre-classical period of yoga, some 5000 years ago in Northern India, was to have a direct experience of the divine. Postural yoga was not emphasized. They practiced meditation, chanting, and various rituals to transcend attachment to the body and to achieve enlightenment. Over time and for a complex set of reasons, including building a national identity during British colonial rule, yoga became a more physical practice. In the late 19th and early 20th centuries, various yoga masters began to travel to the West, and gradually the focus of yoga shifted from a spiritual meditative practice to a physical practice for better health, to maintain youth, and to enjoy a longer life.

But here's the amazing thing about yoga. Regardless of why you start practicing, if you stay with it long enough, you begin to rediscover your inner connectedness to something greater than yourself. Some call it God, others the Universe, and others call it Truth. It doesn't matter what your religious beliefs or affiliations are, or if you are an atheist. Whatever you call this higher power, it is an ideal that lifts you beyond your everyday struggles and helps you clarify, reflect upon, and understand life from a deeper perspective, and to live it more artfully. It is by connecting to this higher state of consciousness that you begin to reconnect to values that express your internal truth, allowing you to create meaning for yourself and to make sense of things.

Yoga takes you into your heart and opens you to tenderness toward yourself and others, teaching you to love yourself and everyone else, warts and all. It teaches you to understand human nature through understanding yourself. It teaches you that you do not see the world as it is; you see it as you are, and that motivates you to want to be your best self. It is a subversive practice that changes you from the inside out, and in due course you become more and more of who you were born to be.

THE EVOLUTION OF SPIRIT

Some time ago I decided to take a year-long meditation course with a renowned yogic scholar as a way of deepening my meditation practice. I was already well grounded in the meditation technique being taught, but I wanted to take a deeper dive into the spiritual aspects of meditation. One of the first commitments we were asked to make was a willingness to engage in sattvic practices throughout the year to support our spiritual growth and development, and to become grounded in the spiritual nature of our meditation practice. We were also asked to write a spiritual autobiography. Yoga tells us that we are spiritual beings having a human experience; that our true identity is eternal spirit. The ultimate goal of yoga is for us to remember that and to become grounded in that awareness. When we identify with our spiritual nature, we can recognize the spiritual nature of all creation.

One of the texts we studied was the *Bhagavad Gita*, part of the *Mahabharata*, an ancient Indian epic poem that tells the story of a family at war, battling for the throne. The Gita, or "Song of God," makes up about 700 verses of the 100,000-verse poem. According to the story, on the eve of battle, Arjuna, the main character, is conflicted about what action he should take. Should he honor his duty as a warrior or as a family member? He agonizes over how he can justify fighting family, some of whom he will undoubtedly have to kill. Feeling helpless and hopeless, he argues that it would be better to forsake his dharma, his duty, and not fight this battle rather than to risk killing uncles, cousins, brothers, his grandfather, or his teacher. He turns to Krishna, the lord, who has been masquerading as his charioteer, for answers to his dilemma. The epic battle is actually an internal one and is an allegory for the moral dilemmas we face on our spiritual journey. Krishna reminds Arjuna that performing his duty as a warrior is his first obligation to fulfill. As part of this conversation, Krishna instructs Arjuna in the three subtle qualities of nature that govern life, matter, and consciousness, and that influence our choices and our happiness. He reminds Arjuna that all objects in nature consist of these three qualities, or gunas, known as: sattva, rajas, and tamas (Easwaran 2000).

Sattva is regarded as the quality of clarity, calmness, and insightfulness. It loves excellence and beauty, and enjoys making the best of whatever it encounters, raising it to a higher level. Sattvic understanding informs us when to act, when to refrain, what is right and wrong action, what sets us free, and what holds us in bondage. Sattvic practices are life-affirming practices that raise awareness and support health and well-being, contentment and joy. When sattva predominates, it manifests as wisdom, reflectiveness, harmony, love, and justice. Sattvic choices can be difficult choices to make as we embark on our spiritual journey because they do not always feel good. But through consistent self-study and emotional balance, we can find our bliss, not as a temporary state, but as the core of our being.

Rajas is associated with the power of action and the energy of intensity. It is willing to push through obstacles to get a result. It loves competing and winning, wants to look good, is not afraid to fight for what it wants, and loves being the center of attention. Rajas can distract us and cause us to lose our inner peace and to look outside ourselves for fulfillment. Any gratification we experience is short-lived. When rajas dominates, it manifests as agitation, turbulence, emotional upset, unreliability, chaos, aggression, or bullying. When balanced, it manifests as courage, passion, determination, and ambition.

Tamas is associated with the state of inactivity. It just wants to rest and escape from having to do anything. It retreats from the world and sleeps, avoids anything that smacks of duty and obligation, or self-medicates to numb out. Its state is heavy and dense, and, when dominant, can manifest as depression, procrastination, apathy, lethargy, addiction, or willful ignorance. When the quality of tamas dominates, we lose awareness of our spiritual nature and we identify primarily with the physical body and all of its limitations. When balanced, tamas can manifest as patience, endurance, and steadiness.

In the yoga tradition, stress and trauma are viewed as an imbalance in the gunas. When viewed wisely as a complete and functional system, we can embrace the gunas and respect their roles in our lives. We need peace to feel safe, we need movement to act, and we need stillness to rest. When we embrace the gunas as useful, with an inclination toward finding balance, we enhance our physical, mental, emotional, and spiritual health and well-being. Sattva is achieved when we combine the energy of rajas with the groundedness of tamas. The goal in yoga is to do just that.

We have considered the psychological impact of ethnic and race-based stress and trauma, and how we in the yoga community can contribute to alleviating the suffering that results. Our focus is intended to be internal. We have discussed what constitutes race-based stress and trauma, how it differs from PTSD, how it impacts our nervous system, where stress and trauma land in our bodies, and what our emotional triggers are. We have explored aspects of cultural conditioning that contribute to racial wounding, and our personal vulnerabilities that make this a difficult conversation. We have imagined what kind of yoga spaces, organizations, and communities we want to occupy and create, and we have explored how Restorative Yoga can be used as an effective self-care tool to buffer the nervous system, increase resilience, and strengthen one's psychological immune system, as we navigate the stresses and traumas that arise from daily lived experiences associated with race. In this chapter we will discuss the role spiritual activism plays in healing racial wounding.

SPIRITUAL ACTIVISM

Spiritual activism is a practice that merges spirituality and activism. It is not about religion, it is not about any form of dogma, it is not an ideology. It is activism that comes not from doing but from the awareness that every moment we encounter is a gift. It is the awareness that you have the opportunity to make every moment that presents itself to you better. Being a spiritual activist means recognizing that every situation you encounter is your teacher and should be met with gratitude and in a spirit of acceptance, compassion, and love. Becoming grounded in your spiritual identity takes practice.

Gandhi, Martin Luther King Jr., Nelson Mandela, and Mother Teresa are examples of change agents who were spiritual activists. What they had in common was consciousness of a power greater than themselves, and they engaged in practices that enabled them to face the storms and problems associated with the work they were called to do. They were doing more than trying to effect external change. They each had internal practices that contributed to their individual personal transformation, and that supported awareness, courage, and stamina. They did more than advocate for change. They practiced change from the inside out by being the change they were advocating for. They demonstrated what they advocated.

Spiritual activism is centered in internal awareness. It is inner-directed and other-focused, asking, "What is the wisest way for me to elevate this situation for the benefit of all?" It is sattvic in nature, balancing rajasic and tamasic energy. It relies on stillness, quiet, and self-reflection before taking action. In moments of stillness and quiet you might be called to action, but this is not the same as reacting to a situation because it upsets you. As long as the thing is freaking you out, whatever it is, you are of no use in dealing with it. The ability to be still in the heat of your own passion without acting, waiting until wise action is revealed to you, is a quality of spiritual activism. Marcus, the man in Chapter 4 who didn't get into a fight with the man who called him an offensive name, or demand retribution by insisting that he be fired, is an example of someone who was able to take an action that was decisive and forceful, but that was balanced. It takes perseverance and dedicated practice to become established in a state of inner calm, but in the end it serves you and all those with whom you come in contact.

Spiritual activism asks you to wait until your inner disturbance passes, allowing you to make peace with the situation in front of you, before you take action. This is true even in emergency situations that require an immediate response. The practice of stillness does not lead to inaction as some might conclude. The practice of stillness with alert awareness leads to wise action. Because Restorative Yoga is practiced in stillness and silence, it helps us cultivate alert awareness and teaches us to listen to our inner wisdom voice before we act.

Activism, peace, and spirituality need to harmonize with each other. If what happens externally creates a disturbance inside of you, it means you are not ready to act from a place of wisdom. When you act from a place of inner disturbance, your actions will reflect that, and in an effort to make yourself feel better, you are more than likely to strike out or turn a blind eye to what is occurring. The problem is, whatever action you take or avoid taking to try to make yourself feel comfortable when you are agitated or disturbed is almost never helpful. External solutions to internal problems do not work. Think about the coffee-shop manager who called the police, the college dormitory student who called the police, and the high school wrestling referee who forced an unnecessary, unwarranted haircut. In their reactivity, they all took actions that made matters worse. Yoga from the inside out asks us to look within before we act out. It is important to ask yourself, "What is disturbing me about this situation?" Then take a moment to let the feeling pass before you take action. Insight and self-regulation are far more effective strategies than acting out of inner disturbance. We are not looking for external solutions; we are looking for inner calm before we take action. Spiritual activism requires a daily practice of meditation, self-reflection, self-awareness, and stillness to balance rajas and tamas to find sattva. This is our daily, moment-to-moment practice. If you do not engage in these practices on a daily basis, you will not be able to call on them when wise action is required. As a colleague points out, the time to teach someone to swim is not when they are drowning.

Spiritual activism starts with acceptance. This is not the same as ignoring a situation. It doesn't mean that you do nothing. It means that your starting position is that whatever is happening is not freaking you out. Once you have accepted a situation, you can see with more clarity because your disturbance is not interfering with your ability to see what is actually occurring. If you are unable to accept that racial and ethnic injustice, inequality, and violence exist, then you will not be able to effectively deal with them when they present themselves. For instance, if someone asks to have a conversation with you about race or ethnicity and you become reactive, or frozen, it means you have some inner work to do to get ready to handle the conversation effectively. Your reactivity, whatever form it takes, is evidence of your own unhealed wounds. Working on healing your own wounds is an important aspect of spiritual activism.

The merger between activism and spirituality comes when you wake up to the reality that you are conscious and aware of what is occurring in front of you, and that whatever it is has nothing to do with what you want, what you planned for, or how you think things should be. This is the starting position of acceptance. The moment unfolding in front of you is the gift being offered you by the universe. Your freaking out does nothing to help. The work is to remain present and not get caught up in the agitation inside of you. The work to do is not in the outside world, trying to get everyone to behave in a way that doesn't upset you, or getting everyone to behave in a way that you want. You will never get things to be the way you want them to be, nor will you ever be able to keep things from being the way you don't want them to be. The good news is that reality is manageable. Understanding and accepting this requires spiritual maturity.

SPIRITUAL DEVELOPMENT

Just as we develop physically, cognitively, and emotionally, we also have the capacity to develop spiritually—to wake up to our naturally loving, joyful, and blissful nature. This is available to everyone, but it requires awareness and a desire to become internally focused and to raise everything to the highest level.

When we are in the childhood phase of our spiritual development, we ask, "What can this practice do for me?" We think that if we meditate, practice yoga, behave ourselves, and follow all the rules, we'll get what we want and avoid getting what we don't want. When that doesn't work, we try harder, or keep looking for the right approach to ensure that we get what we want and avoid getting what we don't want. We remain externally focused and dependent on external solutions to address internal processes. But no matter how hard we try, it never seems to work. Some people remain stuck in childhood spirituality.

In our spiritual adolescence, when we don't get what we want and when things don't go our way, we get mad at the universe, the yoga teacher who betrayed us, the system that betrayed us, the illness we've been diagnosed with, the job we lost, the relationship that ended, or the yoga and meditation practices we have been in engaged in that "didn't work." We are still externally focused, and we act out by rebelling and fighting, or we give up in disgust and frustration and decide, "That's it. I'm done doing this stuff. It doesn't work. It's fake. It's hocus-pocus and a rip-off too. What's the use? What's the point?" We enter a phase of disillusionment because life isn't working the way we thought it did. The methods we were using to have life work out our way failed, and so we get mad at the method and quit our practices. We throw out the baby with the bath water. But disillusionment is a necessary part of spiritual growth. It teaches us that an external focus does not keep life from unfolding in its own way, even if we do meditate or practice yoga. We discover that we are not in charge of life.

If we're lucky, we regroup and turn inward, not to get something, but because we realize that whatever strategy we were relying on before, to ensure that things would go our way, was not necessarily faulty. It was our thought process that was faulty. We thought we could fashion a world to be the way we wanted it to be. Disillusionment is painful but it is a necessary step on the path to spiritual maturity, where you surrender to reality as it is and begin to practice acceptance. This is where we begin to realize that our expectation that life should always give us what we want and work in our favor is the cause of a great deal of our emotional pain and suffering, not just the events that life presents us. This is not to say that when something painful happens, we can avoid being hurt. We cannot. It is to say that the refusal to accept reality as it is adds to an already painful situation and leads to more suffering. With wisdom as our guide, we don't give up our practices. Instead, we honor, accept, and respect what is unfolding in front of us. We do not try to change it. We accept reality as it is, not as we want it to be. This is the starting point of spiritual maturity.

The task is learning to honor and respect each moment, whether we like it or not. This is when we discover that every single moment has something to offer. This is our awakening. Our attitude becomes "I am honored that this is the moment that is presenting itself to me. What is it asking of me and how can I best serve it?" Not "How can I change what is happening, or keep it from happening?" but "How can I serve it?" Anything we do out of emotion or reaction is never the right thing to do. When we don't know what action to take, the central question becomes "Is there something I can do to elevate the situation, not alleviate the discomfort?" In stillness and silence, we can access that information. We just have to be patient and wait for the answer to emerge and for an opening to serve. This is when the situation draws from us what it needs. This is the power of stillness and present-moment awareness.

THE POWER OF STILLNESS

There was once an Indian sage who performed amazing miracles. One day a woman who was deeply distressed approached him. Her daughter was getting married and the family, who had no money, needed 15 grams of gold for her dowry. The sage reminded the woman that he was not a goldsmith, and advised her to sit in stillness, focus on her breath, meditate, and wait patiently for a solution to her dilemma. In the meantime, a wealthy merchant and long-time disciple of the sage approached. He had just been given the news that he was in declining health due to a pre-diabetic condition. He asked for the sage's prayers and blessing. The sage told him to stop eating sugar, and assured him that if he followed this advice, all would be well. In gratitude, the wealthy merchant gave the sage a leather pouch as a gift. Without hesitation, the sage found the woman whose daughter was to be married and gave her the pouch. When she opened it, she fell to her knees in gratitude, for inside the leather pouch she found 15 grams of gold.

Sometimes being still is the most powerful thing we can do. Rather than acting on the advice "Don't just sit there, do something," we are better off taking the advice "Don't just do something, sit there!" This is the path of the peaceful warrior. That is when we discover that just because we're not doing something, it doesn't mean nothing is happening. What is happening is we are getting out of our own way and allowing energy to flow freely through us. As we practice this, the energy blocks that we have created, our samskaras, dissolve. When energy is free to flow, we are able to access our higher-level energy bodies and can act from a place of wisdom and love, those energies that are closest to our spiritual nature.

This is not to say that there is never a time to act. But it is important that we take actions from a place of non-reactivity if we are to be effective. When we react to issues of race and ethnicity from a place of being disturbed by them, we engage in actions to make ourselves feel better and these are usually not actions that are best for the situation. We might cut off a conversation. We might minimize or try to fix a situation. We might ignore it altogether. We might act out in fear or anger and become confrontational or defensive. Being confrontational in response to an offense, or being defensive in response to a confrontation, without any sensitivity or understanding of what needs to be done to raise the situation, might make us feel better in the moment, but none of that is ever helpful to the situation. When we practice being still, we train our nervous system to relax when there is agitation or discomfort and, in the stillness, we begin to notice that the agitation or discomfort dissipates, making room for the energy of wisdom to flow.

We live in a culture that places more value on doing than on being. We attach our worth to our accomplishments. We value how much we do, and how busy we are, more than what we do or how we do it. We miss the point that sometimes doing nothing is more powerful and productive than anything you can do in a situation. But being still is an art that requires practice. It is easier said than done.

Many of us associate being still with being lazy. We consider it a waste of time. Or we may worry that taking time to relax is selfish and end up feeling guilty. Sometimes we are afraid to be still because when we stop filling every moment with activities, we encounter feelings and thoughts we would rather avoid. Sometimes we are afraid to do nothing because our mind tells us we will never be able to realize our dreams if we take time out to be still.

Actually, when you are still, you are better able to quiet your mind and listen more deeply to your heart and soul. It is in these moments that you can hear the still, small voice within that speaks quietly and with confidence from a deeper place of intelligence than your thinking mind. When you act from the depth of your soul and deeper guidance, your actions carry a force and energy that brings you into harmony with life. You will likely find yourself to be the right person in the right place at the right time.

Sometimes you have to slow down so that the world around you can catch up to your vision. There are certain moments in life and situations where there is nothing for you to do but be still. Acting out of impatience will not necessarily make things manifest more quickly but will instead cause you more stress and suffering. Rather than forcing things into existence, slow down, practice being still, silent, and waiting patiently. Connect with the flow of life that already is. Silence has a sound of its own; listen for it. Stillness is just another form of action; revel in it. The real power of living is not just in the actions you take, but also in your stillness. This is not an "either or" proposition. There is a time for doing something and a time for doing nothing.

Use the time you are doing nothing to reflect, restore, rejuvenate, and to prepare yourself for action. If you do not, when the time comes to do something, you may be depleted from all of your busyness and unable to be at your best when it counts the most.

- Learn to trust life.
- Slow down.
- Listen to the silence.
- Enjoy a meditation practice.
- Try Restorative Yoga.
- Don't just do something.

- Sit there.
- Be a human being, not just a human doing.

The work of spiritual activism is to prepare, be calm, and remain open. What do you do if you get dumped on or blindsided? You breathe, you listen, you receive, you hold space for others by just being there, being present, and looking for a moment to elevate the situation. Activism and spirituality are the same at the core level. You work with yourself and come to peace, and if there is something you can do from a place of peace to address whatever is occurring, you can make the situation better because it happened in front of you.

WHEN SPIRIT AND ACTIVISM MERGE

What is the relationship between activism and spirituality? According to Michael Singer, they are the same (Singer 2017). He points out that when we work with ourselves and come to harmony, we are better able to help the situation by making sure that it is better off because it passed in front of us, not by trying to change it to be something else in order to make ourselves feel better. Paying more attention to the spirit in which you act and looking less to the results of your actions becomes your focus.

1. Start with accepting the reality of the situation you are faced with. Deal with it from present-moment awareness. Your preferences and your emotions are irrelevant.
2. Do not waste your time trying to change reality by making whomever is doing what they are doing do something different. It never works.
3. Waking up means acknowledging what is actually occurring and recognizing that you are being asked to honor and serve whatever is presenting itself to you.
4. Instead of wondering why whatever is going on is happening, ask yourself what you can do to make it better, and before you act, wait for an answer.
5. Get centered before you take action. Be still and sit in silence. Wait to see if there is anything the situation requires. If there is something for you to do, it will become clear to you.
6. Listen. Wait for clarity to guide you. This is wisdom.

I will end with two stories both involving Mother Teresa that support the value of stillness and silence and the wisdom of spiritual activism. I don't know if these stories are urban legends or if they are true, and I'm unable to remember where I heard them, but I love them both.

One day a journalist asked, "Mother Teresa, when you pray to God what do you say?" She responded, "I don't say anything. I just listen." "Well, when God talks to you, what does he say?" "He doesn't say anything," she replied. "He just listens, and if you don't understand that, I cannot explain it to you." This is an example of the silent communication that resides within each of us. When we access it, and learn to listen to it, we will be guided to wise action. In another story a journalist asked, "Mother Teresa, do you think it's true that God never gives you any more than you can handle?" She thought for a moment and replied, "Yes, but I wish he didn't think so highly of me."

Make no mistake. The spiritual path is not a pain-free, safe, or easy path. Seeking higher levels of consciousness will call on you to serve in ways that are demanding and sometimes painful. Then, why do it? Because the reward is the experience of boundless joy.

REFLECTION

To Serve with Love

There is a children's story called *The Giving Tree* about a boy who is able to communicate with an apple tree. It begins: "Once there was a tree... and she loved a little boy." In his childhood, the boy enjoys playing with the tree, climbing her trunk, swinging from her branches, and eating her apples. As he grows older, he starts to make requests of the tree. As an adolescent, the boy wants money; the tree suggests that he pick and sell her apples, which he does. As a young adult, the boy wants a house; the tree suggests he cut her branches to build a house, which he does. In middle age, the boy wants a boat; the tree suggests he cut her trunk to make a boat, which he does, leaving only a stump. Finally, the boy becomes a shriveled old man. He wants only "a quiet place to sit and rest," which the stump provides. The story ends, "And the tree was happy" (Silverstein 1964).

As a young mother reading this story to my son, I interpreted its message to mean that giving away everything with no regard for self was the key to happiness. But unlike the giving tree, whenever

I contemplated the possibility of a future as an old stump, it never made me happy.

Most spiritual disciplines teach the virtues of sacrificial love. Setting aside your own needs to meet the needs of another is a beautiful form of love. But taking care of others becomes exhausting and unsustainable if you try to care for everyone else while neglecting your own needs. When the stress of continually being there for others is high, we can become overwhelmed by our own caregiving responsibilities and run the risk of burnout. As I matured, I realized the key to selflessly serving others also involves self-nurturing. Only when we are nurtured is it easy to nurture others. When we do not nurture ourselves, we are unable to draw on the qualities of love and compassion, and other spiritual values that support serving others. Ignoring our own needs renders us unable to give freely from a place of deep caring and compassion. When we give solely out of a sense of duty and obligation, without love and compassion, we feel resentful, taken advantage of, and depleted. In the end, we can wind up feeling bitter and unhappy.

In yoga, selfless service to others is called seva or karma yoga. In her book *The Secret Power of Yoga*, Nischala Joy Devi suggests that to effectively serve others we would be wise to serve ourselves as well. She introduces the practice of karma yoga for oneself. If done regularly, even if only done for 20 minutes each day, self-care can revitalize your body, mind, emotions, and spirit (Devi 2007).

Sometimes we confuse self-care with self-pampering—designer clothes, gourmet dining, extravagant vacations, and other luxuries— or with self-indulgence—spending money you don't have, vegging out in front of your television eating a pint of your favorite ice cream, or catching up on five episodes of your favorite television series. As long as you can afford the luxuries you buy, and as long as you don't make a habit of reducing your stress by choosing quick fixes that don't require much effort, there is nothing wrong with self-pampering or self-indulgence. It's just not the same as self-care.

Self-care, or karma yoga for self, requires effort, focused attention, and perseverance. It means choosing behaviors that balance the effects of emotional and physical stressors. Self-care should balance practices of stillness, exercise, love, and healthy food.

- When you're tired, rest and do practices that will quiet your brain such as meditating, sitting quietly, using positive affirmations, or relaxation techniques.
- Get your life force flowing by walking, running, dancing, doing Tai Chi, or practicing yoga.
- Stay connected. Contact friends at least once or twice a week. Join a book club or a walking group. Be involved in your community.
- Be mindful of what you put into your body, your mind, and your spirit. Make sure your food diet, your thought diet, and your emotional diet are balanced and healthy. Abstain from substance abuse, pursue creative outlets, or engage in psychotherapy.

In the midst of the busyness of life, find what feeds and nurtures you. In order to serve others lovingly, we need to nourish ourselves. When you remember to selflessly serve yourself, service to others comes not from your depth but from your overflow. And when that happens, like the giving tree, you will be happy, even if you are an old stump.

DISCUSSION

- Do you regard yoga as a spiritual practice?
- Do you consider yourself an activist?
- What does spiritual practice involve?
- How do activism and spirituality merge in your life?

REFERENCES

Devi, N.J. (2007) *The Secret Power of Yoga: A Woman's Guide to the Heart and Spirit of the Yoga Sutras*. New York, NY: Three Rivers Press.

Easwaran, E. (2000) *The Bhagavad Gita*. New York, NY: Vintage Books.

Silverstein, S. (1964) *The Giving Tree*. New York, NY: Harper & Row.

Singer, M. (2017) "Bonus Session: Living from a Place of Surrender—The Untethered Soul in Action" [MP3]. *The Untethered Soul, Volume 10: The Power of Inner Clarity*. Sounds True. Accessed on 11/18/2019 at www.store.untetheredsoul.com/audio-lecture-MP3.

Chapter 8

YOGA ON THE MAT

RESTORATIVE YOGA

Restorative Yoga is restful and supported yoga. In this practice, props such as blankets, bolsters, blocks, chairs, neck rolls, and eye pillows are used to support the body in yoga poses, allowing you to come into a state of deep relaxation without falling asleep. Rather than using your own energy, you actually receive energy from the practice and leave feeling rested and refreshed.

For the most part, Restorative Yoga postures are adaptations of traditional yoga postures that are practiced in a deliberately gentler version of the classic poses. Because of the use of props, postures can be held for extended periods of time. Since Restorative Yoga focuses on stress reduction and the release of tension, there is no emphasis on stretching and no reliance on the use of muscle strength in any of the postures. By remaining in the poses for longer periods of time, the actions in a Restorative Yoga practice reach deep into the nervous system, restoring homeostasis, the body's self-regulation system that maintains life. This practice can dissolve chronic tension patterns, and support emotional balance by bringing the body, mind, and emotions back to a state of equilibrium.

Restorative Yoga poses are soothing, as relaxing as a massage, and more restful than a nap. The practice is like pushing a restart button. It is a wonderful self-care tool. Whether you are new to yoga or an experienced practitioner, any body can do it and every body benefits from it. Restorative Yoga helps you learn to rest deeply, relax completely, and rejuvenate physically, mentally, emotionally, and spiritually.

WHEN TO USE RESTORATIVE YOGA

Restorative Yoga postures are ideal for those times you feel depleted or overwhelmed, or are recovering from an illness or an injury. The practice can also help prevent illness and injury by strengthening your immune system, enhancing your awareness, and improving your resilience. Regardless of what other forms of yoga you may practice, how often you practice, whether you are a beginner or advanced practitioner, incorporating Restorative Yoga into your practice once a week, or including a few postures in a daily practice, will help you build up stores of energy that guard against depletion and pave the way for ongoing health.

HOW RESTORATIVE YOGA WORKS

Restorative Yoga is a self-care practice. Stress can overwhelm the nervous system and deactivate the body's ability to heal itself. Your body knows how to function properly and bring itself back into balance. As long as the nervous system is relaxed, the body can be a self-healing organism. Illness and injury can be used as wake-up calls to help you understand what aspects of your life are activating a stress response. Restorative Yoga is a practice that allows you to access your self-healing potential and accelerate the healing process by stimulating the parasympathetic nervous system and restoring homeostasis.

- The use of props minimizes muscular tension and maximizes physical comfort, allowing the body to remain still in postures for extended periods of time.
- Keeping the room dark, warm, and quiet minimizes sensory stimulation and helps soothe and calm the nervous system.
- Keeping the head at or below heart level reduces heart rate, lowers blood pressure, and quiets the nervous system.
- Using diaphragmatic breathing, nasal breathing, and longer exhales lowers heart rate and calms nervous system activity.
- Focusing attention on breath helps evoke the relaxation response.

RESILIENCE

"If it bends, it won't break" is a familiar adage. Resilience is our ability to remain flexible and to adapt to situations and circumstances, as required.

It is essential for recovery from life's inevitable hard knocks. Resilience allows us to bounce back from stressful and traumatic experiences. Being resilient involves being able to tune in to the hidden energy that hides inside each betrayal, loss, heartbreak, and disillusionment we experience. It keeps us from getting stuck in suffering and allows us to use the pain of ethnic and race-based stress and trauma as catalysts for growth. It teaches us to ask:

- What is this situation asking of me?
- What reality do I need to accept?
- What would be the wise thing to do right now?
- What is the gift hidden inside this challenge?

From a yogic perspective, there are three basic building blocks to resilience: tapas, svadhyaya, and Ishvara Pranidhana.

Tapas is a willingness to make the effort to go through hardships and difficulty without avoiding the discomfort such challenges bring. Personal transformation occurs when you are willing to face the discomfort associated with events and circumstances that arise out of your control. This is how we grow and become stronger. Restorative Yoga is an advanced practice that teaches you to be still and silent even in the face of discomfort. It teaches you that sometimes doing nothing is more powerful and productive than any action you can take. It teaches you to reflect, restore, and rejuvenate in order to prepare yourself for action. Tapas is the effort you make to do something whether you want to or not. It cultivates inner discipline. Being still and silent in a Restorative Yoga practice can be challenging. The willingness to do so strengthens you as you remain still and non-reactive through restlessness, boredom, and emotional upheavals that sometimes surface during the practice.

Svadhyaya is a willingness to engage in the practice of self-study to cultivate self-reflective awareness. This requires a willingness to learn from your own life by observing and studying yourself as if you were the most interesting subject on the planet. Self-study is not the same as self-absorption, which is a narcissistic preoccupation with self that disregards others. Self-study is a commitment to knowing the best and worst of oneself, with a desire to recognize how your thoughts, words, and behaviors affect you as well as others. It is the commitment to observing all of this without arrogance or judgment, but with humility for your gifts and with compassion for your flaws. It is the willingness to make changes that will bring you into optimal alignment with what is best in you and best for you and others. Restorative Yoga teaches you how to move through hidden emotional states by remaining aware in the practice of being still, and learning to compassionately observe thoughts and emotions that arise, without reacting to them. When you learn to hold steady in a posture while charged feelings arise, you are strengthening your resilience.

Ishvara Pranidhana is your ability to surrender to reality as it is, not as you want it to be. This ability teaches you to experience the unavoidable difficulties and disappointments of life without constantly wishing things were different. The ability to accept life on its own terms keeps you from feeling victimized, frustrated, and despairing. It is the acknowledgment that there is a higher state of consciousness available to you, beyond the limits of your ego, that can guide, inform, and protect you. When you let go of your need to control reality, you discover that solutions arise spontaneously to seemingly impossible problems. When you align with reality as it is, you open up to love—your highest power. Restorative Yoga provides you with a powerful experience of inner peace and calm. It also offers the opportunity to feel safe in your vulnerability. Knowing that these states are possible gives you the support necessary to get through difficult times.

BREATH

There is a wonderful story in the Chandogya Upanishad 5.1.6–15 about a competition that breaks out between the five yogic senses: mind, breath, speech, hearing, and sight. Each sense maintains that it is the most important of all the senses, and wants to be recognized as such. To discover which of the senses is most important, they decide that each one will leave the body in turn to see who is most missed. Speech leaves first, and although mute, the body lives on. Sight leaves next, and although blind, the body survives. Then hearing leaves, and although deaf, the body perseveres. Next the mind leaves, and although it is no longer very smart, life persists. Finally, breath leaves the body. Naturally, the body immediately begins to die. "Wait! Stop! Come back! Come back!" clamor the other senses. Breath returns to be heralded ever after as supreme among the yogic senses.

This story means to call attention to the breath as the very essence of vitality. It is the animating factor, the conduit of the life force. Without breath, there is no life. The first breath we take at birth indicates that our life has begun. At the end of our earthly existence, we take our final breath. In between our first and last breath, the average person will take about half a billion breaths, but because breathing is something we do automatically and all of the time, unless there is something wrong, it is something we rarely notice. Due to a lack of awareness, we may not realize that our body, mind, emotions, and breath are intimately connected and can influence each other. When we focus on it and control it consciously, breath can provide a link between our conscious mind, our body, our emotional and energetic states, and our spiritual potential.

As we become consciously aware of our breath, we can also become aware that the thoughts we think can influence our breath, and our breath can influence the thoughts we think, as well as our physical body, our emotions, our energy level, and our spirit. Learning to breathe consciously and with awareness is an essential tool for our sense of well-being.

DIAPHRAGMATIC BREATHING

Diaphragmatic breathing, a form of deep breathing, is an important tool that is used in Restorative Yoga to help us relax, restore, and maintain balance in our mind, body, emotions, energy levels, and spirit. A regular practice of this type of deep breathing can:

- reduce anxiety
- lower/stabilize blood pressure
- increase energy levels
- relax muscles
- decrease feelings of stress and overwhelm.

Diaphragmatic breathing reverses stress in your body by stimulating the main nerve in the parasympathetic nervous system, the vagus nerve, slowing down your heart rate, lowering your blood pressure, and calming your body, mind, and emotions.

When you breathe diaphragmatically, instead of using the muscles in your neck and chest, you are using your abdominal muscles and your diaphragm. By breathing diaphragmatically, you are conditioning your respiratory muscles and improving the efficiency of oxygen exchange with every breath. This allows more air to flow into your lower lungs. It also reduces strain on the muscles in your neck and upper chest, giving them a chance to relax. Diaphragmatic breathing is more relaxing and efficient than chest breathing, allowing higher volumes of oxygen to reach the body's cells and tissues. Diaphragmatic breathing reverses physical stress in your body and helps slow down emotional turbulence in your mind, making you less reactive to events and to your emotions.

Three-part breath helps train the muscles in your diaphragm and abdomen to open up, allowing the lungs to take in more oxygen. It relieves stress and tension by stimulating the parasympathetic nervous system. It eases emotional distress, leading to a sense of calm, and improves concentration in preparation for meditation.

You can choose to step more deeply and purposefully into the process of your own breath at any time or any place. To do so is, literally and metaphorically, to choose to participate more fully in life. Virtually every yoga tradition is intent upon cultivating a more conscious relationship with the breath.

Enjoy your breath. Your breath is the voice of your body. The quality of your breath is what determines whether or not it is pleasurable. Your breath has a story to tell. When you listen to your breath, you become attuned to its messages. When it speaks to you in whispers, like a soft lullaby, soothing and rocking you in its warm embrace, it calms you. When you feel agitated, breath is labored and turbulent, moving rapidly with intensity. Breath's movements rhythmically ebb and flow like waves in the ocean. Pay attention. Each inhale and exhale tells a story of the natural ebb and flow in all of life. Breathing easily and fully is one of the basic pleasures of being alive. The breath holds the secret to the highest bliss. It is the dominant factor in the practice of yoga. By listening to the breath, we are able to receive its blessings. When we practice being still and silent with awareness, we are able to receive, reflect on, and enjoy our breath. This is one of Restorative Yoga's greatest gifts.

The illustrations in this chapter are available to download in color from www.jkp.com/catalogue/book/9781787751859.

DIAPHRAGMATIC BREATHING TECHNIQUES
THREE-PART DIAPHRAGMATIC BREATHING

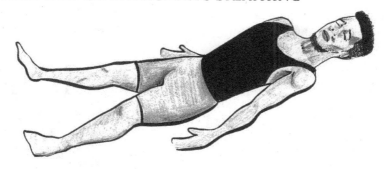

Begin by lying on your back in the relaxation posture, on a flat, carpeted surface or your yoga mat. Support your head and neck with a thin blanket, or a rolled-up hand towel, or a neck pillow placed in the curve of your cervical spine. Your chin should be lower than your forehead, which lengthens your neck and calms your mind. Extend your legs long in front of you. Let your feet fall out to the sides of your mat. Place your hands, with your palms facing up, a few inches away from your body, or place one hand on your belly and one hand on your heart. Your eyelids should be gently lowered or closed. Close your mouth as you breathe through your nose. Stretch your body long on the ground and let go of any tension. Release and relax your whole body. Focus your awareness on your breath.

1. Inhale fully through your nose, keeping your belly soft and feeling it rise. Feel the breath enter the bottom of your lungs, then fill the middle of your lungs, then fill the top of your lungs with breath.
2. At the top of your inhale, hold the breath to a count of three, while keeping your body still, before you begin your exhale.
3. Exhale slowly through your nose to a count of six, emptying your lungs from top, to middle, to the bottom of your lungs; hold your exhale out to a count of three before beginning your inhale. Feel your belly move in toward your spine.
4. After you complete one full cycle of three-part breath, return to your normal rhythmic breath without holding the breath in or out for three full inhales and exhales, then return to the three-part rhythmic breath for two more cycles. Now resume seamless rhythmic three-part breathing, without holding the breath in or out, for 5–15 more minutes.

SEATED DIAPHRAGMATIC BREATHING

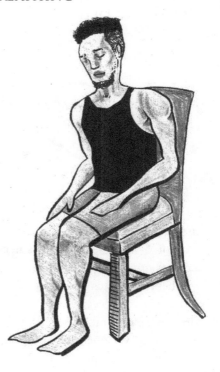

Sit erect in any seated pose. If you are seated in a chair, plant your feet firmly on the ground and sit so that your shoulders are over your hips, your ears are aligned with your shoulders, and your chin is parallel to the ground. This ensures that your spine is erect. Place your hands, palms down, on your thighs, or place one hand on your heart and one hand on your belly. Close your eyes, or lower your eyelids, and begin to focus your awareness on your inhalations and exhalations. Soften your belly and the sides of your rib cage. Keep your spine erect and let the muscles of your back support your posture without effort. Notice how your breath fills and expands the sides of your rib cage and the front of your abdomen. Keep your belly soft. Continue to observe your breath until its pace and depth feel comfortable and relaxed. To support the stimulation of the parasympathetic nervous system, inhale to a count of two and exhale to a count of four. Seated diaphragmatic breathing helps maintain equilibrium in challenging situations, reduces everyday levels of stress, and helps you focus your mind with greater ease. Do this several times until you begin to feel relaxed and then resume your normal pace of breathing. This practice can be done for 5–20 minutes.

CROCODILE POSE—MAKARASANA

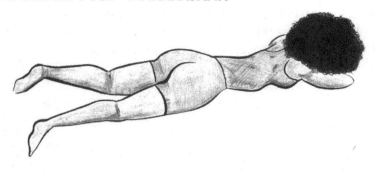

Lie on your stomach with your arms folded at a 45-degree angle above your shoulders. Rest your forehead on your folded arms, or prop your upper body with a cushion or folded blanket, with your chin draped over the cushion. Turn your feet in with your legs close together or out, separating your legs until your thighs rest on the floor. Your body will naturally begin to breathe diaphragmatically. Bring your awareness to the movements of your belly, the sides of your rib cage, and your lower back. Notice how the belly expands and presses against the floor as you inhale and slightly lifts, moving in toward your spine, as you exhale. Notice how your ribs expand out as you inhale and move inward as you exhale. Notice how your lower back rises and expands as you inhale and falls as you exhale. Feel the movement of breath around the entire torso—front, sides, and back body. Remain in this pose for 7–10 minutes. Come out of the posture slowly and resume normal breathing. This practice can be done for 5–20 minutes. Crocodile pose deepens the breath and eases the normal abdominal tension that occurs when you are nervous or anxious. It aids in breathing more naturally.[1]

SPINAL HEALTH

One of the most important structures in the human body is the spine. Your backbone is what holds you upright. While the spine is doing its work to hold you up, gravity is doing its work to hold you down, causing compression in your spine. Compression builds up tension around the

---

1   This is not recommended for women who are more than three months pregnant.

spinal column as the body attempts to hold itself upright. This can cause muscle spasms and muscle fatigue.

When the spine is properly aligned, gravitational forces flow easily through it. Alignment occurs when the curves of your cervical, thoracic, lumbar, and sacral spine are balanced in relationship to one another. The spine is a communication conduit for the brain, transmitting signals that affect movement, breathing, sensation, and mood. When the curves of the spine are balanced, each curve transitioning smoothly into the other, messages from the brain are communicated through the nervous system in a clear and coherent fashion. This balance offers optimal support for overall health and well-being. Lifestyles that involve sitting hunched over computers, bending to get in and out of cars, sitting for long periods of time behind the wheel of a car, slouched on the couch watching television, and sleeping on mattresses that are too soft make you prone to misalignments, which, over time, can cause gradual degeneration of the structure of the spine, compromising your overall health. The good news is if you regularly engage in balanced movements that maintain the integrity of the spine, these misalignments can be corrected. Restorative Yoga can help with that.

Breathing plays an important role in spinal balance. The mechanics of breathing help move your spine in ways that support alignment. When you focus your awareness on your breath and exercise conscious control of your breathing, you can become aware of the movement of your spine as your breath guides it. The movement of your spine with your breath is the same in all positions. The wave of breath moves your spine like an accordion. With each breath your spine grows longer and then releases. Depending on the position you are in, the elongation and release of your spine might occur when you inhale or when you exhale. When you observe what your breath is inviting your spine to do, and just allow it to happen without trying to control the natural movement that occurs, you will notice that the release of your spine comes through your willingness to surrender and relax, rather than through using willpower or effort.

By observing that your breath moves your spine, you begin to shift your awareness from an external focus to an internal one. As this shift occurs, you are able to see how your body, mind, emotions, and breath are linked and how you respond to the movement that is taking place. A balance of ease and effort is needed to honor the relationship between your breath and the movements of your spine.

In order to maintain a healthy spine, you need to move your back for brief periods of time each day. Moving the spine in all possible directions is a way of maintaining flexibility and mobility. Your spine can move in five directions. It elongates, folds forward, bends backward, lengthens sideways, and twists. A balanced Restorative Yoga practice will likely include a combination of spinal movements; however, just using one of the poses that moves the spine out of a neutral position each day is a good way to keep your spine supple, flexible, and aligned.

RESTORATIVE POSES

Restorative Yoga is a self-care practice that supports stress reduction and can aid in recovery from trauma. It is well established that trauma and stress are not just mental constructs, but actually exist in the body. The body has an awareness that is deeply visceral, different from cognitive awareness. Restorative Yoga supports embodied awareness, which is awareness that reaches deep into the nervous system, where contracted states caused by stress and trauma can release. This is where profound and lasting change takes place.

The poses being suggested support embodied awareness and enhance an overall sense of well-being. Ease is emphasized in this practice to evoke the relaxation response, which aids in rest, repair, recovery, and resilience. The postures, done with the support of props, and held for extended periods of time, counteract fatigue, energize, relax overall muscle tension, restore homeostasis, and support emotional balance. In this practice, first you find the form of the pose and then you make any adjustments that are necessary to make yourself as comfortable as possible.

The suggested poses are illustrated to give you a visual example of the form, accompanied by a description of how to get into the posture. Once you have found the form of the pose, make whatever adjustments you need to make so the pose is as comfortable as possible. The props are used to support you so that you do not have to stretch or use any muscle energy. Covering yourself with a blanket for warmth is important as your body temperature will likely drop as you come into deep states of relaxation. You may find that you need to use more than the minimum number of props suggested, or you may need fewer than the suggested number to be comfortable. This is your practice. Remember, in this practice you want to experience ease. Your body will tell you what is optimal. You do not have to put up with any discomfort whatsoever. Let common sense guide you in your selection of poses. Some may be more comfortable and more beneficial than others.

INVERSION
LEGS UP THE WALL—VIPARITA KARANI

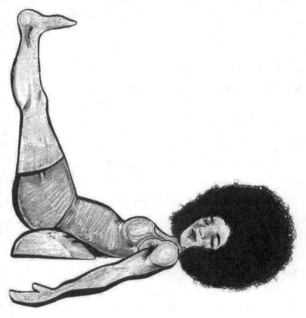

To perform this receptive inversion, start by sitting on the floor against a wall, knees slightly bent, feet flat on the floor with your right shoulder, hip, and thigh against the wall. Place your hands flat on the floor hip distance apart and slightly behind your hips, fingers facing forward. Begin to lower yourself onto your back, bending your elbows back behind as you swing your legs up the wall. Once your legs are up the wall, scoot your hips as close to the wall as is comfortable. Keep a bolster, or a folded blanket in a rectangular shape, within reach. Bend your knees, press the soles of your feet into the wall, lift your hips, and slide the bolster or blanket underneath them. Straighten your legs and extend them back up the wall. Extend your arms out to the sides, palms facing up, if comfortable, or place your arms in cactus position. If you choose cactus position, lift your arms out to the sides of your body in the shape of a "T" at shoulder height. Bend your elbows to

90 degrees. Keep your upper arms horizontal and bend your forearms back behind you until the backs of your hands are flat on the ground.

If extra support is needed, place a small neck roll (made from a hand towel, for example) under your neck to support and lengthen the cervical spine. Rest in this pose for up to fifteen minutes. When ready, bend your knees and press the soles of your feet into the wall and lift your hips to slide the bolster out from under you. Gently lower your pelvis to the floor, and with knees still bent, roll to the right side, walking your feet down the wall, coming into a fetal position. Pause, enjoy your breath, tuck your chin, and use your hand to press yourself back up to sitting.[2]

ELONGATION
SUPPORTED RESTING POSE—SAVASANA

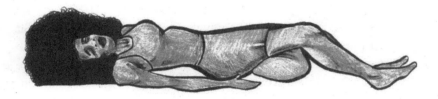

Sit on the floor with your legs slightly bent. Slide a bolster or blanket roll beneath your knees and slowly lower your back, neck, and then head onto the floor. If your cervical spine needs support, place a small rolled-up hand towel or neck roll in the curve of the cervical spine to lengthen it, then place your head on the floor. Let your arms rest comfortably by your sides, preferably palms facing up to broaden and place your shoulder blades more squarely on your back. Close your eyes or use an eye pillow if you are comfortable doing so. Become aware of your natural rhythmic breath, and let go of any tension you may feel. Rest here for 5–20 minutes. When you are ready to come out of this pose, roll onto your right side, coming into a fetal position; pause here, take two or three breaths, tuck your chin into your chest, and gently press your hands into the floor to lift back up to sitting.[3]

---

2   This is not recommended for women who are on their moon cycle or after the third month of pregnancy.

3   This is not recommended for women who are more than three months pregnant.

SIDE LENGTHENING
SUPPORTED SIDE BEND—SUPTA ARDHA CHANDRASANA

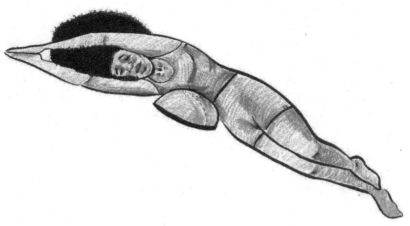

Place a bolster or a blanket roll horizontally in the middle of your mat. Sit with your right hip against the short end of your bolster or blanket roll; your legs are softly bent behind you with one leg on top of the other. Place a square folded blanket, block, or pillow between your knees, and lean to the right. Place your right hand across the top of your bolster toward the far side of your mat and lower down over the bolster onto your right side. Once lowered onto the bolster, extend your right arm straight along the ground with your palm facing up and rest your head on your biceps. Extend your left arm straight up overhead with your palm facing the short edge of the mat. Lower your arm over your ear until both right and left palms touch. Feel the length in your left side body. Observe your breath and notice how it guides the movements of your spine as you lengthen and release. Relax your entire body and pay special attention to your neck and side body as the breath circulates from front to back and around your rib cage. When you are ready to switch sides, slowly turn your body face-down, pause, enjoy your breath, and then gently press your hands into the ground to rise up. Repeat on the other side. Hold on each side for 2–10 minutes. When you are ready to come out of this pose, take two or three deep diaphragmatic breaths, tuck your chin into your chest, and gently press your hands into the floor to lift back up to sitting.[4]

---

4   If you are more than three months pregnant, instead of lying across a bolster, lie on the left side of the body, in a fetal position.

FORWARD FOLDING
CHILD'S POSE—BALASANA

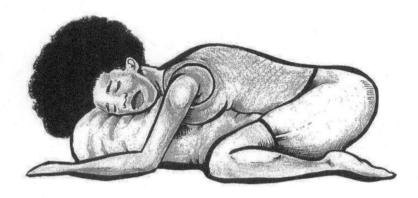

Create a support of firm pillows, blankets, or a bolster lengthwise on your mat in front of you. Lower onto your hands and knees, placing them on either side of the support, knees open wide toward the edges of your mat; the tops of your feet are flat on the floor behind you with big toes touching. If needed, place a folded blanket under your knees or under the tops of your feet for comfort. Sit back onto your heels and, without lifting your hips, fold your torso forward over the length of the bolster or blankets. If your hips are tight, lift up and place a bolster or blanket roll under your hips or behind your knees for support. Place your forearms and the palms of your hands flat on either side of the bolster, or, if it is more comfortable, bend your elbows and interlace your fingers around the top edge of the support. Turn your head to one side or the other, resting on your cheek, or rest your forehead on the bolster—whichever is most comfortable. Let gravity pull your legs and hips toward the earth as you soften your lower back, and release your tailbone toward your heels. Halfway through, turn your head to the other side as your body continues to settle into the pose. Hold this pose for 5–10 minutes on each side. When you are ready to come out of this pose, take two or three deep breaths and gently press both hands into the floor to lift up to sitting on your heels.[5]

---

5   This is not recommended for women who are more than three months pregnant.

WIDE-LEGGED SEATED FORWARD FOLD—UPAVISTHA KONASANA

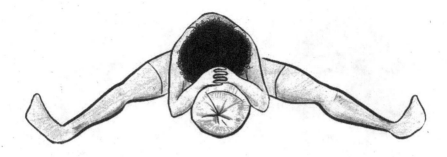

Sit on a blanket folded into a rectangular shape facing the long side of your mat and open your legs to a wide V position. Place the narrow end of the bolster between your legs. Fold forward from your groin, not your waist, and rest your forehead on the bolster. You should feel your legs and back body lengthening but not stretching. Use as much elevation on top of the bolster as you need to keep from over-stretching in this forward fold. You can do this by placing as many blocks as you need on top of the bolster for a head rest as you come into the forward fold. Your range of motion will determine how high your support needs to be. Rest your forehead on the support or turn your head to the side and rest your cheek on it. Use a square folded blanket or a rectangular folded blanket to cushion your head if you like. Rest your arms on either side of the bolster or drape them over the top. Hold this pose for 5–10 minutes. When you are ready to come out of this pose, tuck your chin into your chest, and lift your torso to an upright position, remove the bolster, place your hands behind your knees, and gently lift them until your feet are flat on your mat.[6]

---

6   This is not recommended for women who are more than three months pregnant.

SUPPORTED FACE-DOWN RELAXATION POSE—DOWNWARD-FACING SAVASANA

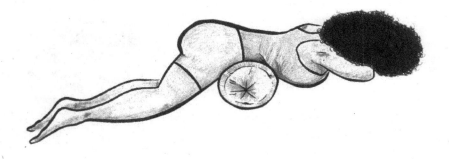

Place a bolster, rectangular folded blanket, or rolled blanket horizontally across the middle of your mat. Facing the top end of your mat, kneel at the bolster or blanket. Position your hips at the bolster or blanket and lay your torso across the top so that your hips are raised on it. Extend your arms forward with bent elbows and place one hand on top of the other, creating a cushion for your head. Lower your forehead onto your hands or turn your head to one side, resting on your cheek. Let your legs and feet relax, and let your heels fan out toward the outer edges of your mat while your toes turn in. Hold this pose for 5–20 minutes. Focus on your breath. When you are ready to come out of this pose, press your hands into the floor and, with your chin tucked, lift yourself back off the bolster or blanket, and come into child's pose with your arms draped horizontally over the bolster. Hold here for at least five full diaphragmatic breaths and then lift up to sitting.[7]

---

7   This is not recommended for women who are more than three months pregnant.

SPINAL ROTATION
SUPPORTED SIDE TWIST—SALAMBA BHARADVAJASANA

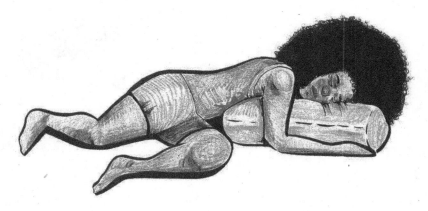

Place your bolster or three rectangular folded blankets stacked on top of each other vertically in the middle of your yoga mat. Sit with your right hip snug up against the narrow end of the bolster. Bend both knees, taking your shins to the left and resting your left ankle in the arch of your right foot. Lift up from your sternum and twist your belly toward the right to square your torso to the front of your mat. Fold over the bolster from this position. Rest your right cheek on the bolster so that your head is facing the same direction as your knees. Keep the back of your neck long and the front of your neck soft. Rest your forearms and hands along the sides of the bolster. Now notice how your breath slows down and deepens. Observe how your inhalations and exhalations root your pelvis and enhance the turning sensation in your belly and shoulders. Do you root more deeply into your pelvis when you inhale or when you exhale? Do you lengthen and move deeper into the twist when you inhale or when you exhale? When you are ready, change sides. Hold this pose for up to 15 minutes on each side. When you are ready to come out of this pose, press both hands into the floor, tuck your chin into your chest, and come up to sitting, lifting your head last.

BACK BENDS
SUPPORTED BRIDGE POSE—SETU BANDHA SARVANGASANA

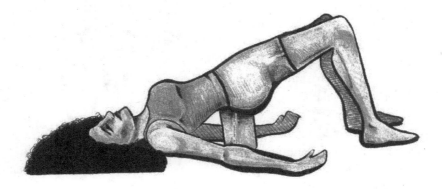

Lie down on your mat. Bend your knees with your feet flat on the mat about hip distance apart and about six inches from your buttocks. Lift your hips, and place a block, bolster, or folded blanket under your hips. Choose the height that feels best under your lower back. Remember that comfort, not intensity, is key. Lower your hips onto the prop you have chosen. Relax with your arms extended along the sides of your body and your palms facing up, or in cactus position. If you choose cactus position, lift your arms out to the sides of your body in the shape of a "T" at shoulder height. Bend your elbows to 90 degrees. Keep your upper arms horizontal and bend your forearms back behind you until the backs of your hands are flat on the ground. Focus your awareness on your breath. Remain in this pose for a minimum of three minutes to a maximum of ten minutes. When you are ready, lift your hips, remove the prop, and lower yourself to the floor. Roll onto your right side, coming into a fetal position, and rest here for 5–10 full breaths. Tuck your chin into your chest and use the strength in your arms to lift up to sitting, with your head following last.[8]

---

8   This is not recommended for women who are more than three months pregnant.

SUPPORTED RECLINING BOUND ANGLE POSE—SUPTA BADDHA KONASANA

Place a bolster or a narrow stack of three rectangular folded blankets vertically in the middle of your yoga mat. Place an additional folded blanket or a neck pillow at the top of your bolster to support your head or your neck. The lower edge of the blankets or bolster should come directly into contact with your buttocks to support your lower back. Bring the soles of your feet together, touching as if in a prayer position, and spread your knees apart. Each knee fanned out to the side is supported by a yoga block, blanket roll, meditation cushion, or bolsters. Lower yourself onto your back over the bolster. If you like, cover your eyes with an eye pillow and cover your body with a blanket. Breathe deeply and surrender to gravity as you relax. This pose should be held for a minimum of 5 minutes and can be held for up to 20 minutes. To come out of the pose, put the soles of your feet on the floor, bend your knees, and roll off the bolster onto your right side, coming into a fetal position. Pause there for 5–10 breaths and enjoy your breath. To come out of the pose, tuck your chin into your chest and use the strength of your arms to lift into a sitting position.[9]

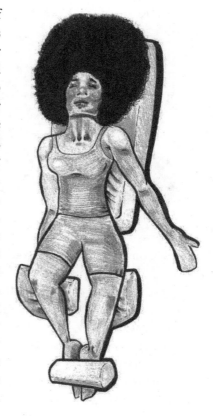

9   This is not recommended for women after the third month of pregnancy unless a block is placed underneath the bolster at the top of the bolster, raising it to a slant and elevating the torso and the head.

MEDITATION
WHAT IS MEDITATION?

Meditation is a practice that trains the mind to focus internally so that it becomes more than just a storehouse of information but is cultivated as a tool of awareness. Meditation is the observation of the mind. It is the ability to notice your thoughts, and your emotions, without analysis, while sitting in stillness and silence. A meditative mind is not necessarily a quiet mind; rather, it is an observed mind.

WHY MEDITATE?

Meditation brings clarity to your thought process. When you sit to meditate, you are inviting the mind to come to stillness, and you are teaching the mind that you are in charge of it, not the other way around. At first your mind will wander off in any direction it wants, but over time, with consistent practice, the mind will come to stillness for brief periods of time. Meditation cultivates awareness of your inner world, your inner voice, and allows you to see with more clarity, less judgment, and less constriction. It takes you out of your analytical mind and into your intuitive wisdom. Meditation helps cultivate wisdom consciousness through self-study and offers you the direct experience of your higher levels of consciousness. Meditation requires:

- attention or gentle awareness
- focus
- willingness to do it.

WHAT TO EXPECT

- It is natural to have thoughts in meditation. Thinking is what minds are designed to do. In meditation do not try to control your thoughts. Instead, observe them and let them go.
- Focus your attention. When you close your eyes or lower your eyelids to meditate, you have a focus. It could be your breath, a mantra, or an object such as a candle.
- The process of meditation involves interrupting the constant flow of thought with your focus. When the mind wanders off, gently

invite it back to the focal point. You are training your attention to focus on one thing at a time.

- When you realize you are daydreaming or involved in a thought that has entered your mind, gently refocus. Rather than reacting, in meditation you are continually returning your attention to the object of your focus.
- When your mind comes to stillness, your body relaxes. When your body relaxes, it involuntarily releases stress. The stress release can come as a thought, a memory, an image, flashes of color, an involuntary sensation or movement, or an unexpected emotion. Do not become distracted by any of that. Simply return your attention to your focal point.

The content of your thoughts or other experiences you may have in meditation are unimportant. It does not matter why you thought the thought, remembered an event, felt what you felt, or saw what you saw. Stress is being released. As stress is released, we feel calmer and are able to see with more clarity.

MEDITATION GUIDELINES

- Do not try to meditate. Just do it with intention, not effort. There is no goal to achieve. Release all expectations.
- Be kind to yourself. How you treat yourself in meditation is how you treat yourself in life. Be sweet to yourself. This is a powerful yet benevolent process.
- Stay in the process and stick with the practice no matter what. Trust that whatever does not nourish you is released—a visual, an emotion, or a thought. Do not cling or avoid. Even if you are restless and bored, you have had a good meditation. You cannot judge the quality of your meditation by your experience during meditation.

THE BENEFITS

Meditation results in clearer thinking. Self-reflection with a clear mind takes you beyond having to learn everything from firsthand experience.

It removes you from relying on pain as your best teacher and offers you wisdom instead. It teaches you to rely on your own awareness and your intuitive understanding. It teaches you to pause before acting on your impulses, which reduces reactivity. You become more peaceful and calmer. You are better able to regulate your emotions, focus your attention, and make clear choices. People who meditate regularly tend to have less anxiety and stress, are better able to notice negative thinking, are better able to concentrate, feel more compassion, are more creative, have improved memory, and emotional balance is restored.

IDEAL DAY MEDITATION

Begin your day with this meditation, ideally after brushing your teeth and taking your shower, before you eat, preferably at the same time each day, prior to any other activity. Select a dedicated quiet space free of clutter and distractions, and take a comfortable seat.

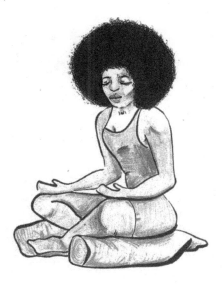

Close your eyes and focus your attention on your breath. Notice the coolness of your breath as you inhale and the warmth of your breath as you exhale. Continue to observe your breath for several rounds. When you feel ready, ask yourself how you would most like to feel as you go through your day, regardless of what occurs. Do not try to think of a response. Wait for one to spontaneously emerge to the level of your conscious awareness.

Once the feeling has revealed itself to you as a thought, a feeling, a sensation, a memory, or a visual image, focus your awareness on what arises and then think the word that describes it. Silently repeat the word as your mantra, allowing the feeling to fill your consciousness. On your inhale let the feeling fill you from head to toe. On your exhale let the feeling surround you. At the end of seven minutes invite your awareness to return to the surface level of consciousness. Before you open your eyes and begin your day, sit in stillness for at least one minute.

You can do this more than once a day if you like, but stick with the feeling that first made itself known to you in the morning. If it is the second or third time you have used this meditation in one day, just sit in stillness and silently repeat the word for 3–5 minutes.

YOGA NIDRA—DEEP REST

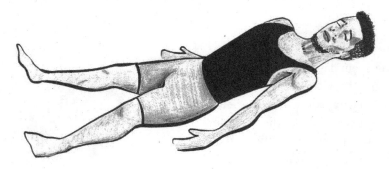

INSTRUCTIONS

Yoga Nidra is also called yogic sleep. It is a practice that takes you into a deep state of relaxation that approximates sleep, but, unlike sleep, you remain conscious as you move deeper into a dream-like state. The following exercise is a variation of Yoga Nidra and is not meant to take you into a yogic sleep, but involves bringing your attention to your body, part by part, as you move into deeper states of relaxation. A complete session of Yoga Nidra can take more than an hour but you can try this version for as long as it takes to go through each body part and to then return your focus to your breath.

Lie down using any props you may need to support you in being comfortable. If lying down is not possible, sitting in a comfortable chair with a straight spine will do. Once you are comfortable, close your eyes or lower your eyelids and shift your awareness to an internal focus. Become aware of your body and notice how it feels. Massage your fingertips with your thumb tips. Notice the feel of your body as it rests on the ground or on the chair. Notice the feel of your clothing as it caresses your skin.

Systematically, go through each body part, being very specific. Take your time. Relax your scalp, your forehead, and your face. Release any tension in your eyes, your cheeks, your mouth, and your tongue. Relax your entire face. Lengthen the back of your neck by slightly lowering your chin. When you get to your arms and legs, relax each side of the body separately, first one side and then the other. Beginning on your right side, relax your arm, then your hand, and relax each finger one at a time. Relax your right shoulder, then your upper back, your middle back, and your lower back. Relax your diaphragm, and your belly. Relax your right hip, thigh, knee, calf, ankle, foot, and then relax each individual toe on your right foot. Shift your attention to the left side of your body and repeat the entire process, beginning with your left arm, hand, each individual finger, your left shoulder, and your upper, middle, and lower back. Continue inviting your awareness to travel all the way down the left side of your body in the same way you did on your right side. Let go of any remaining tension and let your body be soft and open.

Notice the sensations of your breath. As you breathe through your nose, feel the sensation of coolness in your nostrils when you inhale. Notice how your belly softens and expands, and how your chest rises as your lungs fill with breath. Feel the sensation of warmth in your nostrils as you exhale, and notice how your chest deflates and your belly moves in toward your spine. Bring your attention to the space where your inhalation meets your exhalation. Notice the gap between each breath. Your breath is in the present moment. Fill your lungs with breath and feel the fullness and nourishment each breath gives you. Now inhale to a count of three and hold your breath to a count of three. Then exhale to a count of three and, at the bottom of your exhale, hold your breath to a count of three. Do this for five full rounds of breath, and then return to your normal rhythmic breath. Remain here, focused on your breath until you feel finished.

Slowly bring your awareness back to the surface level of consciousness and let your awareness rest here for two or three minutes before you move on to your next activity. If you are on your back before you sit up, role to your right side, coming into a fetal position, tuck your chin into your chest, and use the strength of your arms to return to a sitting position.

RESTORATIVE YOGA: A SOUL-CARE PRACTICE

This book has emphasized that yoga is more than a physical practice. It is a practice that involves body, mind, emotions, and spirit, bringing all aspects of being into harmony. As such, the practice of yoga speaks to the very heart and soul of our being. It is more than a self-care practice. It is a soul-care practice. Here are some suggestions for enhancing your practice that you can try both on and off your yoga mat.

STILLNESS: Inner stillness connects us to our intuitive wisdom and guidance and helps us make better choices. Stillness practices can include meditation, Restorative Yoga practices, sitting in silent prayer, sitting and listening to music, or sitting quietly in nature. Schedule time each day to quiet your mind and relax your body. Start with something small. Do the Ideal Day Meditation for seven minutes each day. Add a restorative pose to your asana practice. Journal. Breathe deeply for a few minutes. There are many ways to practice being still and they do not have to include going on retreat or sitting in silent meditation for hours. Begin and end each day with a stillness practice.

ORDER: Whether you are aware of it or not, order, harmony, and balance are a reflection of serenity and are a reflection of a calm, peaceful mind and spirit. When things are out of place, it can be jarring to the nervous system. It is easier to relax, restore, and rejuvenate in an ordered environment. Order your environment each evening before going to sleep and wake up to an uncluttered, peaceful space to begin your day. Something as simple as making your bed and tidying up before you begin your daily routine can do wonders to calm you. Start each day anew.

UNLEARN: We have all been conditioned to see the world a certain way, and after a while our perceptions become habits. We fall into the habit of thinking that our way of seeing is the only way. To see the world with new eyes, we have to break out of habitual ways of perceiving. This involves what I refer to as unlearning. Unlearning requires mindfully paying attention to the ways we have always thought or behaved, to determine if our habitual behaviors are relevant to the situations we presently face. If not, a period of unlearning precedes learning to make way for new thoughts and behaviors. As a simple example, learning that you have thoughts but that you are not your thoughts usually requires some unlearning. Recognizing that just because you are doing nothing does not mean nothing is happening usually involves some unlearning. Unlearning that hard work is not necessarily your best work is another example. Examining what one has learned about race and ethnicity usually involves some unlearning before real change occurs. Unlearning involves recognizing the perceptual filter through which you are seeing. Then realizing that there are more ways of perceiving reality than your own. When you take the seat of the observer, you are able to see that your response is one of many possible responses. With this insight, you have the choice to cling to the old habitual way of responding or to experiment with a new response. This is how we grow.

LOVE: Community and group support are vital to health and well-being. We are meant to be with each other. This is especially true during and after times of stress. But don't wait for a stressful event to connect with others. Contact your friends regularly, preferably in person or by phone. Reach out to others. Offer your gifts and talents. Create communities of the heart.

CONNECTION: The purpose of yoga is to connect yourself to your highest nature—inner peace, tranquility, wisdom, and love. We do this in our yoga practice on the mat by linking breath to movement, heart to mind, and off the mat by linking heart to heart.

AWARENESS: Your mind is more than a storehouse of information. It is also a tool of awareness. There is something beyond thought, beyond emotion, beyond speech and action. It is a place of awareness. Taking the seat of awareness allows you to notice your thoughts and emotions without acting on them. Instead, you pause, reflect, and then choose. This is freedom.

RESILIENCE: This is the ability to recover and bounce back from adversity, an unexpected or unwelcome change, and to grow from the experience.

EVOLVE: Where there is life, there is change. Without change, there is no growth and no life. Reflect on change, its inevitability, and how to gracefully accept it, even if it is uncomfortable. The ability to embrace change is an essential part of living. To align with life, you must be one with change and "go with the flow."

CREATING YOUR RESTORATIVE YOGA CLASS
WELCOMING ENVIRONMENT

Create a welcoming holding environment so people have an opportunity to feel safe in your presence, in the space, in their body, in their spirit, in their core, and in their vulnerability. This is done by bringing caring attention to each one of your students. A caring environment is a prelude to holding a wider range of human experience. Arouse friendliness, warmth, and tenderness in your students by modeling it yourself. This helps keep wholesome states of mind around and unwholesome states of mind at bay. Orient toward the positive and resist mixing the positive with the negative. You want to address the unsettledness of the person walking into the room. Friendliness filled with affect is what constitutes a safe holding space. A welcoming environment arouses self-compassion, curiosity, a sense of wonder, and wholeheartedness in your students. Orient toward comfort in the body first, then in the mind.

AMBIENCE

The room should be dark, warm, and quiet. The nervous system responds to these cues by relaxing. As the students relax and blood pressure lowers, body temperature drops. The room should be at around 80 degrees Fahrenheit (27 degrees Celsius), and blankets should be available to cover students for more warmth. Eye coverings are optional. Some students, particularly those who have experienced some form of trauma, may be averse to closing their eyes or having them covered. If you offer eye covering, always make it optional. Your students will tell you whether or not they want to close their eyes or have them covered. Eye covering can support relaxation and should be made available for those who choose it. Music is optional, but sound, even ambient sound, can be distracting. Rather than relying on music, use your voice as a musical instrument. When you speak in prosodic tones, it is very comforting and aids in evoking the relaxation response.

MOVEMENT

The primary movement in this practice is the breath. Other than transitions to the next pose, the body remains still throughout the practice. If there is fidgeting during the practice, it is a sign that there is some discomfort and an adjustment might be called for.

ADJUSTMENTS

In this practice, first you find the form of the pose and then you make whatever adjustments are needed to make the experience more comfortable. It is important to articulate this to your students. Finding comfort is not something people who are chronically stressed or traumatized do, so this is an important emphasis. If the student asks for help, or you observe that the student is clearly not able to make an adjustment without assistance, approach them carefully and quietly, synchronize your breath with theirs, then gently make a suggestion that will support more ease in the posture. It is important that the student has his or her own experience without unnecessary input from the teacher. Once the adjustment has been made, ask the student how it feels. Always take your cues from the student.

SEQUENCE

Create a sequence that flows easily from one posture to the next so as not to disturb the peacefulness being cultivated with unnecessary movement. Less is always more in a Restorative Yoga practice. Three to four poses are optimal for a 60-minute practice, and sometimes even that may be too much movement. The more experienced you become in teaching Restorative Yoga, the more skillful you will become in determining how much is too much. Choose a balance of poses that move the spine in various directions. If you choose three postures, include a forward fold, a twist, and a backbend. If there is time, you can also include an inversion to reverse the flow of gravity.

PROPS

Use props to support the body for maximal comfort. The recommended minimum number includes: one bolster, two blankets, two blocks, cushions, or pillows, one eye covering, and one neck roll. In a Restorative Yoga practice you cannot have too many props—the more, the better. If you do not have access to props, the poses can be practiced without props, but will not be as comfortable. Shorter holds is one way to modify a practice without props. This is a practice that emphasizes stillness, ease, and comfort, an important experience for people experiencing ongoing, recurrent, cumulative stress and trauma.

ORDER

The room should reflect peace, calm, and order. If you set the room up for your students, which is frequently done in workshop settings, blankets, bolsters, blocks, and any other props you may be using should be placed neatly next to the yoga mats. If students are setting up the room themselves, instruct them in placing their mats, blanket folding and prop placement. For ease of use once the asana practice begins, blankets should be folded in half vertically, then folded in half horizontally, then folded in half horizontally again. The blanket will be rectangular in shape, making it easy to use in a variety of ways. Teaching blanket folding and prop placement brings awareness to how a neat and ordered environment can be soothing and relaxing. By the end of the practice, of course, the room will undoubtedly be in disarray!

Once the room is set, state your theme for the class. Relying on the yamas and niyamas as your guide will help you develop themes that address important aspects of the yoga practice. Next, introduce the postures. End the class by asking students to share one word that describes how they feel.

VOICE

Use your voice like a musical instrument. Use a tone that is soothing, calming, clear, firm yet gentle. Your voice is an instrument of healing. Be mindful of your pace and your delivery. Be measured in your delivery. There is no hurry. Let silence work for your students. This is a practice where the less said, the better.

RHYTHM

Be mindful of the pace of your delivery. Be slow and methodical. Set your instructional rhythm to your most comfortable relaxed breathing pattern.

SILENCE

Rely on silence as your teaching assistant. Silence speaks to your students and allows them to have their own experience and to hear their own inner voice. Silence teaches your students how to listen to their inner wisdom.

LANGUAGE

The way you use language is critically important. Invite students to go deep into their experience of breath, body, space, stillness, busyness, contraction, expansion, and present-moment awareness. Use language that invites them to trust their own experience, that arouses a sense of wonder, curiosity, playfulness, gratitude, and interest. Be mindful of the language you use to instruct. Make sure your instructions are clear and inviting.

All yoga postures have a beginning, a period of transition, and an end. Here are some examples of how you might phrase your instructions:

1. To begin: "When you are ready…" followed by clear instruction.
2. To transition: "Stay here if you like, but if you are ready to move to the next posture, (name it), take a deep inhale through your nose, and exhale through your mouth."
3. To end: "Come into a fetal position, pause, be aware of your breath, notice what you feel, tuck your chin, and use the strength in your arms to come up to sitting." Set up the next pose.

The best way to learn to teach Restorative Yoga is to incorporate restorative poses into your regular practice schedule and spend at least 20 minutes in the practice, as it usually takes that long for the mind and body to come to rest. Explore stillness and quiet in the practice mindfully. As you engage in the practice, you become your own best teacher. This is also what you want for your students. Include a variety of poses in the practice that move the spine in different directions: forward, sideways, backward, and an inversion or an elongation are your choices. A well-rounded practice might include three postures in whatever combination supports your theme. For example, a supported forward fold, Balasana; a supported side twist, Salamba Bharadvajasana, or a supported side-lengthening pose, Supta Ardha Chandrasana; a supported backbend, Supta Baddha Konasana, or an inversion, Viparita Karani. Experiment with how you begin and end each practice, but ending with a supported savasana is familiar and soothing. At the end of each practice remember to invite your students to share one word that describes what they are experiencing. This anchors what they have experienced with an awareness of its impact.

Frequently Asked Questions

How often should I practice Restorative Yoga?

You can practice as often as you like. Some people practice daily, especially when they are faced with emotionally or physically challenging circumstances. Others find that a once-a-week practice is sufficient to help them maintain equanimity. For those who enjoy an active practice, including one or two restorative poses in the practice is enough.

How is Restorative Yoga different from Yin Yoga?

Restorative Yoga involves no stretching, whereas Yin Yoga involves holding the body in stretching positions for extended periods of time.

How is Restorative Yoga different from a gentle Hatha, or slow flow yoga?

All forms of yoga can be restorative, but Restorative Yoga is practiced in stillness and silence, with props to support the body, with only three or four poses in a 60-minute class.

Can Restorative Yoga be taught without props?

Props support the body in feeling comfortable and relaxed without distraction. If there are no props available, as is sometimes the case, the poses described can all be done without props, but will probably not be held as long. The emphasis should be on comfort, stillness, and silence within the practice. Sometimes imagining that you are resting on props helps when none are available.

Should I make physical adjustments?

Fidgeting indicates discomfort. Approach the practitioner quietly; synchronize your breath with theirs first. With permission, a gentle touch to calm agitation is sometimes enough. If it is not, quietly ask if you can make an adjustment by raising, lowering, adding, or removing a prop. Once you have made an adjustment, ask how the practitioner feels.

Should I use a timer in my meditation?

Using a timer can be jarring to the nervous system. If you want to know how long you have been in meditation, there is nothing wrong with opening your eyes to check the time and then returning to your meditation if you want to continue.

Will Restorative Yoga make me too relaxed to get anything done?

I once had a student tell me that she couldn't risk practicing Restorative Yoga because all she wanted to do after the practice was take a nap. If you worry about becoming too relaxed, because you have something important to do, only do a 10–20-minute practice that will energize and refresh. If you find that after an extended practice you need more rest, this suggests that you are probably sleep-deprived and would do well to get more rest in your daily life. Going to bed the same day you get up is a good place to start. In other words, go to bed before midnight. This may require some lifestyle changes, but if that leads to better health and well-being, it is worth it.

Afterword

SELF-STUDY

Yoga involves more than the physical practice of asana. It includes lifestyle practices designed to align us physically, mentally, emotionally, and spiritually. It is holistic. An important practice in the yoga tradition is svadhyaya or self-study. It involves the cultivation of self-reflective awareness. One aspect of self-reflective awareness is a psychological process of turning within to observe your mental and emotional state, to notice how your mind processes thoughts, feelings, sensations, and experiences, and to examine your past history in order to learn from it. Psychological self-study usually involves some form of analysis to make meaning of what one has observed or experienced. Questions that surface during this form of self-reflective thought might include "Why did I do, say, or think that?" "What does it mean?" "Why does that bother me?" "What does it have to do with my past?" There is a reliance on the thinking mind to gain insight, to find answers, and to interpret meaning. While psychology originally meant the study of the soul, it has come to mean the study of the mind. The problem is that our analysis and interpretations, both functions of the thinking mind, are based on our conditioning and our perceptions, and are not reflections of a deeper reality beneath the surface of thought. The thinking mind does not always get things right. It fluctuates and makes mistakes because of a variety of influences that interfere with clear, non-biased perception and awareness.

In the yogic tradition, self-study practices go beyond observing personal thoughts, emotions, and sensations and examining past history, all of which are aspects of the conditioned individual self. Yoga asks us to take a deeper dive into the fundamental nature of consciousness itself. It tells us that consciousness is not something that happens in the mind. It is not something we are producing, it is not personal, and it does not exist inside of you. You live inside of it. According to the yogis, the substance of each individual self is embedded in and is an aspect of infinite consciousness, the source of all being. In ancient times, svadhyaya, self-study, consisted of engaging in practices that imprinted the idea of infinite consciousness on the mind over and over and over, until individual awareness and infinite consciousness merged. Svadhyaya asks us to let go of who we think we are so that we can discover more of who we truly are. Its fundamental question is "Who am I?" In moments of illumination, the self is experienced as the underlying foundation of our individual awareness. As the experience of our individual self changes, we see things differently because new perceptions become available to us.

Practices of meditation, reading inspirational and sacred texts, chanting and mantra are examples of activities that cultivate this level of self-reflective awareness. But any activity you are engaged in that supports self-reflective awareness can become a self-study practice. The activity will be different for different people. But this is what all compassionate self-study practices share: the commitment to observing one's self without interpretation or analysis, arrogance or judgment, expectation or attachment to any outcome. In compassionate self-study we observe ourselves with humility and compassion, for the purpose of cultivating higher levels of consciousness that will bring us into alignment with our core nature. Studying ourselves in this way requires cultivating a discipline of loving kindness toward ourselves. By observing ourselves through the eyes of loving kindness, we open the way to learning from our own lives. By studying ourselves lovingly and respectfully, without shame, blame, or criticism, we access our own internal guidance system and discover not only that are we our own best teacher, but that we are also our own best student. Life itself becomes our classroom. We discover that we can learn from our successes as well as from our mistakes.

Our closest relationships can be wonderful vehicles for mirroring important aspects of ourselves, and can take us into deeper contemplation of those parts of self that may have eluded us. At times that means being open to receiving compliments about traits and qualities that reflect what is best in us. At other times we may receive feedback that invites us to consider making some changes. Regardless of its nature, feedback always provides us with an opportunity to go beneath the surface into a deeper contemplation of self.

You are bound to become more self-aware when you choose a path of self-study. By deepening your commitment to the practice, you can begin to observe your mental, emotional, and spiritual misalignments without shame, blame, or criticism. Even if it is uncomfortable at first, self-study creates an opportunity to make adjustments in your thinking and behavior that can bring you into alignment with what is best in you and optimal for you. This can greatly enhance the quality of your life, benefitting you and all those around you.

WHAT DIFFERENCE DOES A DIFFERENCE MAKE?

In the Introduction, I told stories about certain race-related events that were emotionally painful. I was not always able to handle the emotions that arose in me without reacting. Sometimes I would cry, sometimes I would rage, sometimes I would fall into depressive states. The practice of yoga and meditation, plus life experience and maturity, taught me how to remain non-reactive. Being non-reactive is not the same as being passive or indifferent. Rather, it means feeling what you feel and waiting until the emotion passes before taking action, to allow a creative response to emerge and guide your behavior. I can honestly say that after years of practice I am rarely triggered any longer to the point of being hijacked by my emotions when old wounds surface, or when new ones are sustained. My hope for you is that you are willing to take a deep dive into the exploration of your relationship to your own race and ethnicity, and then go deeper. As I mentioned in the Introduction, I do not know what difference, if any, my attendance at a racially segregated university made to those whom I encountered while I was a student, or to those who came after me. By the same token, I have no way of knowing what difference this book will make, but what I do know is this: if it helps one individual engage in the work of self-discovery, then this book has served its purpose.

I will end with one final story. You may have heard it. There are many versions of the story, but in the one that was told to me, a man is walking on a beach after a storm where there are thousands of starfish that have washed ashore. As he walks, the man notices a child picking up one starfish at a time and throwing it back into the ocean. He watches for a while and then asks the child, "What are you doing?" "I'm cleaning up the beach and saving all the starfish." "But there are thousands of starfish on the beach. Throwing one starfish at a time back into the ocean can't possibly make any difference." The child smiles, picks up another starfish, throws it back into the ocean and says, "It makes a difference to this one."[1]

The starfish story is a story about making a difference. What difference are you trying to make? You do not have to change the world to make a difference. The challenge is to recognize that by doing your own inner work, you are making the biggest difference of all. This is change from the inside out.

There is a prayer I like to share with my students to remind them of where and how real, lasting change begins. I call it the Serenity Prayer Re-mix.

> *God, grant me the serenity to accept the people I cannot change*
> *Courage to change the one I can*
> *And wisdom to know it's me.*

Change the world by changing yourself. Become the change you want to see. That is how you will make a difference.

Peace and blessings to you on your journey.

---

1 Adapted from Loren C. Eisley, *The Star Thrower*, A Harvest Book, Harcourt, Inc. Orlando Austin New York San Diego London. Copyright 1978 by the estate of Loren C. Eisley.

Subject Index

abhinivesha 139
acceptance 168, 170
acculturation 124–5
activism (spiritual) 166–9, 173–4
adaptive responses (unhelpful) 103
adjustments to pose 205
ahimsa (non-harming) 148
aloneness 115–6
anamaya kosha 100
anandamaya kosha (bliss body) 100–1
anandamaya kosha meditation 101
ancestral memory 56–8
aparigraha (non-attachment) 153
appropriation 150
asmita (ego) 137–8
asteya (non-stealing) 149–50
attachment (raga) 138
attitudes (unconscious) 140–1
attuned relationship 78, 84, 85, 96
autonomic nervous system (ANS) 84–5
aversion (dvesha) 138–9
avidya (misapprehension) 137
awareness, place of 203

back bends
    reclining bound angle pose 196
    supported bridge pose 195
Balsana (child's pose) 191
Bhagavad Gita 164–5
"Blind Man and the Elephant" parable 52–3
blind spots (cultural) 128–36
bliss body (anandamaya kosha) 100
blocked energies 106

body/mind/heart alignment
    99–101, 113–4, 202–3
brahmacharya (moderation) 151–2
breath
    essential nature of 181
    and spinal balance 186
    utilization of 48, 112
    see also diaphragmatic breathing
bridge pose (supported) 195

change, surrendering to 153
child's pose (Balasana) 191
Clarks' research 31–2
class environment
    ambience of 204
    facilitation of incidents in 55
    order in 202, 206
    welcoming 204
coffee shop arrest 51–2, 63, 90
color blindness 130–1
colorism 133–4
comfort zone (expanding) 111–3
communication, silent 174
communities of care
    creating 159
    definition 143–4
    yoga communities 144–6
connection 73, 203
consciousness 211–2
contentment (santosha) 155, 160–1
context, importance of 51
Crocodile pose (Makarasana) 185
cultural blind spots 128–36

AUTHOR INDEX